The Ultir
to Surrogacy
& Home Insemination

Barrie Drewitt-Barlow

To

Taylor e Simon

Good luck e Best wishes !

Brrie x

The Ultimate Guide Company

2011

First published in Great Britain in 2011 by The Ultimate Guide Company, 30 City Road, London EC1Y 2AB.

British Library Cataloguing in Publication Data. A catalogue record for this book is available from the British Library.

ISBN 978-0-9569919-0-4

Printed and bound in Great Britain by CLE Print Ltd, Huntingdon, Cambridgeshire.

Photographs courtesy of Sarah Pallett, Bourn Hall Colchester.

Contents

Acknowledgements

This book is the culmination of 14 years in the world of surrogacy, first as an Intended Parent and then as a coordinator of surrogacies. During this time I have been lucky enough to meet some of the world's leading fertility experts, and to work with them to provide a first-class service to those wanting to start a family with the help of a Surrogate Mother or Egg Donor.

Special thanks to the following:

Anthony Drewitt-Barlow, for the past 24 years the love of my life, who never gave up on me or on our dream of having a family. He put up with my constant moaning and groaning, and one failed embryo transfer after another; he stood by me until we had our family. I thank you.

Our children Aspen, Saffron, Orlando, Jasper and Dallas, all born through the help of Surrogate Mothers and Egg Donors.

Dr Guy Ringler, CFP Los Angeles. After six failed embryo transfers and four failed egg retrievals at another fertility clinic, Dr Ringler was going to be our last hope. He certainly was! Special thanks and much love and respect to a fantastic man.

Rosalind Bellamy, our first Surrogate Mother and the Birth Mother to our first set of twins, Aspen and Saffron.

Donna Calabrese, our second Surrogate Mother and the Birth Mother to our third child, Orlando, and our second set of twins, Jasper and Dallas.

Tracie, Biological Mother and Egg Donor to three of our children, and our second Egg Donor Andrea.

My publisher, Linda Riley of The Ultimate Guide Co.

And finally to the team at The British Surrogacy Centre in Maldon, Essex and San Francisco USA, who spend 20-hour days working to help create families through surrogacy.

This book is dedicated to everyone who wants to have a child of their own, and in particular to the thousands of couples who have been through years of infertility issues, miscarriage, and in some cases the loss of their child too.

Foreword

Surrogacy has helped many thousands of couples and singles who would never have had the chance to parent otherwise. For my partner Tony and I, our journey is complete, and five children later, born through surrogacy, we are complete. Surrogacy has given us the family we so wanted, and has opened up the world to Alternative Families.

After years of trying to adopt and foster in the UK, Tony and I decided that the only way forward for us to have a child together was to go down the surrogacy route. People say there's a reason why things don't work out; ours was so we could have our own biological children. As much as I would have loved to adopt a child, there is nothing better than having a child who is biologically yours. But maybe one day, now that we have our own biological children, we may be lucky enough to welcome a child into our home who has come to us via adoption too.

Fourteen years on, and now with five children born with the help of Surrogate Mothers and Egg Donors in the USA, our family is complete (or is it?). In any case, the fact remains: without the help of surrogacy, we would not have our beautiful family now. During our journey I have been active in the surrogacy community, offering support to others in the same way that we received support ourselves. Early on I also decided to 'go public', and during years of being featured in the print media alongside worldwide TV appearances, I have highlighted both the positive and negative sides of surrogacy. As a social worker by profession, I also realized the need for professional information and support, and this led to the opening of the British Surrogacy Centre, the first centre in Europe dedicated to facilitating surrogacy and offering practical advice on home inseminations.

This book is the culmination of the experiences that we have been through as a couple struggling to have a family of our own, along with my professional experience assisting others to do likewise. I wanted to share our personal experiences of our journey, away from tabloid interpretations, and to provide you with the facts. The aim of the book is to give you a clear understanding of how the process works, and what Intending Parents need to consider when going through the journey. Addressed to Intending Parents, the book will also be of interest to professionals, family members and friends.

Wherever you are on the journey as an Intending Parent, this book will answer your questions and guide you through the maze of dos and don'ts that are the downfall of so many couples going through the surrogacy process. Among other issues, you need to be fully aware of the cost and legal implications, and you should use this book as a tool to guide you to the right people to help you. The people and organizations that I recommend in this book are known to me personally. I have either worked with them myself, or I feel they are the best in their chosen fields because of the reputations that they have built up over many years.

However, I must stress that it is still important for you to vet every service provider you work with, to ensure that you are getting the right service and advice for *you* to ensure you have a smooth surrogacy journey. Good luck!

Barrie Drewitt-Barlow

1. What is Surrogacy?

Surrogacy is an arrangement in which a woman carries and delivers a child for another couple or person. The woman may be the child's genetic mother, or she may carry the pregnancy to delivery after having an embryo to which she has no genetic relationship transferred to her uterus. There are different ways to arrange surrogate pregnancies, and various procedures available. If the pregnant woman receives financial compensation for carrying and delivering the child (besides medical and other reasonable expenses), the arrangement is called a commercial surrogacy. Otherwise, the arrangement is sometimes referred to as an altruistic surrogacy. Altruistic surrogacy does not involve any financial agreement: for example, when a sister or other relative carries a baby for the Intended Parents.

The Intended Parents (that is, those who intend to raise the child) may arrange a surrogate pregnancy because of infertility or other medical issues that may make a pregnancy or delivery impossible, risky or otherwise undesirable. An Intended Parent could also be a single person or a same-sex couple wishing to have their own biological child. Over the past ten years, an increasing number of same-sex couples and single people have turned to surrogacy to help start their family.

The first mention of surrogacy was in the Bible:

"Now Sarah, Abraham's wife, bore him no children and she had a handmaid, an Egyptian, her
name was Hagar. And Sarah said unto
Abraham, 'Behold now, the Lord hath
restrained me from bearing: I pray thee, go
unto my maid: it may be that I may obtain children by her.' And Abraham hearkened to the
voice of Sarah." Genesis 16:1-2

Surrogacy first started to became commercial in the
United States, in the late 1970s. It has been estimated
that between 1976 and 1988, 800 babies were born to
Surrogate Mothers. This number of surrogate births
soared to 7,000 in the following four years, as infertile
couples found it to be an ideal way to have children.
The number of surrogate births has continued to rise
since then, and is currently estimated to be up to
40,000+.

Today, infertility is a growing problem, with one in
eight couples having difficulty in conceiving, and one
in seventeen couples being unable to conceive after
two years of trying. Fertility treatments have offered
hope to many, but the sad truth is that many of these
fail. More and more same-sex couples, too, are considering starting a family now that their relationship and
family structure are recognized by the law. It is unsurprising that surrogacy is coming to be widely regarded
as a mainstream alternative to childlessness.

We live in an age where we have the technology to
be able to build a family regardless of our infertility
issues. When carried out in an ethical way, surrogacy is
most definitely the way for you to have the family that
you have always wanted. Ensuring that you are as fully
informed as possible before beginning, and that you
are working with the right team of people, will enable

the process to run smoothly for you and to give you the family that you want.

Types of Surrogacy

There are two main types of Surrogacy: Traditional and Gestational. Once you are in possession of all the facts, the type you decide to opt for has to be a personal preference, as both have their advantages and disadvantages. Either way, apart from in a tiny minority of cases you will be working with a commercial Surrogate. This is a Surrogate who requires a 'base fee' (USA) or 'expenses' (UK) that are above and beyond the actual amounts you would have paid out if you were able to carry the baby yourself.

While finding an altruistic Surrogate (most likely a family member or friend who will not take one penny from you other than actual expenses) is almost impossible, finding a commercial Surrogate will be relatively straightforward.

Traditional Surrogacy

For many years, Traditional Surrogacy used to be the only way for a couple to use a Surrogate. This method uses the egg of the Surrogate Mother and the sperm of the Intended Father. Fertilisation can be performed in an IVF clinic, but more often the technique of Artificial Insemination happens at home. (See Chapter 4. for more details.) In this situation the baby is biologically related to both the Intended Father and the Surrogate Mother.

Pregnancy using a Traditional Surrogate is much like any other pregnancy, without the injections and other medications required in Gestational Surrogacy. When the baby is born, the situation is handled similarly to an adoption, where the Traditional Surrogate will sign over her parental rights to the Biological Father and Intended Mother. This is complicated in some countries, including the UK, by the fact that, if the Surrogate is married at the time of giving birth, her husband is regarded as being the legal father of the baby. (This is discussed in detail in Chapter 8.) This is why most Intended Parents seek a Surrogate who is not legally married during their pregnancy, as the hope is that the Surrogate will put down the Intended Father's name on the birth certificate.

There have been many cases over the years where couples have entered into arrangements with Surrogates to carry the biological baby of the father and the Surrogate. In these cases no legal adoption or placement has ever had to be granted by a court, as custody is simply regarded as being a casual arrangement by the biological parents. In the UK, a biological father named on the birth certificate now has just as many parental rights as the mother, and the baby can legally live with him with the agreement of both parents.

As I have said, these types of arrangements have been happening for many years now. For those who are cost conscious, it is still something that happens a lot in countries like the UK, where fathers have these rights. However, there are still many pitfalls with these types of arrangements. The first and most overwhelming consideration is the fact that the Surrogate is still and will always be seen as the child's mother in terms of legal parental responsibility. As such they will maintain certain parental rights over the child until the child comes of age.

Of course, in most cases this is not going to matter to most of the people in this kind of set-up, purely because they have all become good friends by now and are happy with the arrangement. However, this is not true in all cases. In fact, several have become nightmares for both the Intended Parents and the Surrogates. Cases include Surrogates changing their minds at the birth — or even before the birth in some cases — and cases where the Intended parents have also changed their minds and left the child with the Surrogate. There have also been cases of Surrogates wanting to become too involved in the parenting of the child more than a year after the birth.

Most recently in the UK, there have been cases where the Surrogate has changed her mind, and then gone after the Intended Parents for Child Support payments. So not only have the Intended Parents' hopes of a family together come crashing down around their heads, they are also now stuck with this other woman in their life, who they have to pay a significant amount of their earnings to each month to support her and the baby she was carrying for them.

The warning here is that you really do need to do your homework. Don't be tempted to take the cheaper option simply because it is cheap, and don't agree to go though your surrogacy with someone you have only just met in the pub because you feel she is your only option for having the family that you so desperately want.

It is also extremely important with Traditional

Surrogacy arrangements that there should be NO sexual intercourse involved. This would invalidate the process of surrogacy in the UK for the purposes of the application for a Parental Order. (The Parental Order in the UK, once granted, allows for the name of the Intended Mother or other Parent to be used as one of the child's official parents, and that name can then be placed on the new birth certificate.)

What are the advantages and disadvantages of using a Traditional Surrogate?

One advantage of Traditional Surrogacy from the Intended Parents' perspective is the relatively low cost. Artificial insemination is less expensive than In Vitro Fertilization (IVF). There is no egg donation fee, which will save many thousands of dollars. It is usually less medically complex, which also means fewer costs for the Intended Parents. In addition, if the first effort at Artificial Insemination does not work, then a second try can be made within weeks, rather than waiting months as is usually the case with IVF. And from the Surrogate's point of view it is a speedy and painless process, and the Surrogate seldom needs to take fertility medication.

However, although Traditional Surrogacy is the simpler of the two types of surrogacy in as much as conceiving is less complicated, mentally it can be the hardest to accept. There are many who believe that the downside to Traditional Surrogacy is the genetic link between the Surrogate and the baby that she carries. It is not just more difficult for the Surrogate Mother to give up her own biological child; it is also harder for the

Intended Mother to accept a child that her husband has fathered with another woman.

However, many women who do choose to be Traditional Surrogates describe their feelings on the matter as being similar to egg donation. I personally find this strange, because the Egg Donor simply donates her eggs after a relatively short period of some 15-20 days, whereas the Traditional Surrogate is carrying a baby who is genetically linked to her for up to nine months. Some would argue that the feeling of parental bonding must be there between the Surrogate and the baby at some level; that after months of the baby moving, the scans, the sitting and touching of the belly, there must be something that Traditional Surrogates feel that contributes to the bonding process.

There are also those Intended Parents who worry about the legal ramifications of Traditional Surrogacy. In US case law, for example, the Courts have rarely (if ever) favoured a Gestational Surrogate in the very few cases where a custody dispute has arisen, but have been more likely to side with the Surrogate when she is the genetic mother of the child that she has carried. In the few cases of Traditional Surrogacy that have come to the courts in the UK, the court has always sided with the Surrogate. At the time of going to press, we have not yet seen a dispute between a Gestational Surrogate and Intended Parents go to a UK court, so the predicted outcome in these cases is unclear.

Traditional Surrogacy is typically used today by couples or singles who might have been offered the services of a close friend or relative who they trust completely. Most Intending Parents these days are more inclined to go down the Gestational route to create their family, because they feel that the chances of a Surrogate changing her mind is less.

I personally am not a fan of Traditional Surrogacy, and would encourage those who can to go down the Gestational Surrogacy route. I do understand that this type of surrogacy has worked for many years for lots of people, and it is certainly a cost-effective way of creating a family through surrogacy. However, for those of you who do choose to take this route, PLEASE follow the rules; it will save you many problems in the long run. Get legal advice as soon as you know your Surrogate is pregnant, so that you can put the right things into place when the baby is born to establish you legally as the parent.

Gestational Surrogacy

Gestational Surrogacy uses In Vitro Fertilization (IVF) to create an embryo using the ova (eggs) from the Intended Mother or Egg Donor and sperm from the Intended Father or Sperm Donor, after which the embryo is implanted into a Surrogate. This process allows the Intended Parents to have a genetically related child wherever this is possible. In either case, the child has no genetic link to the Surrogate. Intended Parents might use Gestational Surrogacy for a number of reasons, such as when the Intended Mother is unable to carry a pregnancy safely and successfully, or when the Intended Parents are unable to produce ova/eggs or sperm, or when embryos fail to implant in the Intended Mother.

It is important to remember with surrogacy that you are NOT dealing with infertility. In most cases, you are going to use the egg of a twenty-something-year-old woman (if you are using an Egg Donor), and the uterus of a woman who has had no infertility issues in her life and has had, in most cases, several successful pregnancies prior to being a Surrogate for you. The likelihood is that your Surrogate is going to get pregnant so long as you use the right clinic and method to achieve a pregnancy.

In my view, Gestational Surrogacy is the best way forward for many couples who have been fighting infertility, and for same-sex male couples. It takes away the fear that the Surrogate will have a legal case to keep the child if you do have a breakdown within the process that leads you all to the court room. In the USA, you would also be able to establish your rights as the Intended Parents within the contract you set out with your Surrogate before the medical procedures took place. You would be able to establish parental responsibility in a court room during the pregnancy, well before the birth of the baby takes place.

In the UK, where Surrogate contracts are not deemed to be legally binding, these will still show courts that the intention at the start of the process was for one woman to carry the biological child of another set of parents to term, because for whatever reason they couldn't.

The term Gestational Surrogacy actually describes several variations in surrogacy:

Gestational Surrogacy using the Intended Mother's Ovum (Egg) and the Intended Father's Sperm

This type of Gestational Surrogacy uses the Intended Mother's ovum (egg) and the Intended Father's sperm, with a Surrogate carrying the baby to term. This requires the Intended Mother to be able to ovulate and produce viable eggs.

The clinic will check the viability of the Intended Mother to produce her own eggs by running an AMH (AntiMullerian Hormone) test, which can be performed any time during her menstrual cycle, followed by an FSH (Follicle Stimulating Hormone) test on day three of the cycle (or of the next cycle depending on where she is in her current cycle when she first goes to see the clinic). Both tests can normally be coordinated to take place within the first week of a cycle, so that as soon as a woman starts to menstruate, she would call the clinic and arrange her first appointment.

This method is used by heterosexual couples when, for whatever reason, the female partner cannot carry a healthy pregnancy to term even though she is fertile. In Vitro Fertilization (IVF) techniques are used to retrieve the Intended Mother's eggs, and subsequently to fertilize them with the Intended Father's sperm. One or more of the resulting embryos are then transferred to the Surrogate's uterus. Any remaining embryos are then frozen for subsequent attempts or for siblings.

Gestational Surrogacy Using Donor Ovum (Egg) or Sperm

Another form of Gestational Surrogacy uses donated eggs and/or sperm. This happens when the eggs and/or sperm of the Intended Parents are of poor quality because of illness or advancing age; or where a single person or same-sex couple want to start a family. The donated egg is fertilized with the Intended Father's or donated sperm, and after the embryo has grown in the laboratory for a few days, it is implanted in the Surrogate's uterus.

As with all forms of Gestational Surrogacy, there is no genetic link between the Surrogate and the child who she carries. The ethnicity or colour of your Surrogate will have no bearing whatsoever on the outcome of these areas on your baby.

For example, in my own case, all five of our biologi-cal children are white Caucasian, born with blonde hair and either blue or green eyes. However, our Surrogates are both of different races to us. Rosalind, our wonder-ful first Surrogate, is Mexican, and our wonderful second Surrogate Donna is mixed-race Japanese/white European. None of our children bear any resemblance whatsoever to either women, but bear a striking resem-blance to their Egg Donors. (They do, though, have very strong likes and dislikes food-wise that reflect their Surrogate Mothers' dietary preferences during the pregnancies. Aspen and Saffron are absolute lovers of Mexican-style foods, while Orlando cannot get enough of Sushi and other food stuffs that Donna liked!)

There are a large number of Egg Donors available across the UK and US, although as payment for eggs is not permitted in the UK as it is elsewhere, it tends to be a little harder here to find available donors. Each individual country or State has their own law governing egg donation, and especially the financial implications; see Chapter 8 for further details about surrogacy/egg donation and the law.

What are the advantages and disadvantages of using a Gestational Surrogate?

In both these types of surrogacy, the Gestational Surrogate (also known as the gestational carrier) is unrelated to the child. In general, it has been seen over many years that this approach works best for the Surrogate, the Intended Parents, and most importantly, the child.

Laws about Gestational Surrogacy vary from place to place. In many parts of the world it is still not legal to pay a Gestational Surrogate, although the couple who hire her may pay for her healthcare and compensate her for expenses related to the pregnancy. You also have to remember that contracts for surrogacy arrangements are not always enforceable in every country around the world, or in fact in every State in the US, even when surrogacy itself is legally recognised.

The legal status of the baby also varies. As with Traditional Surrogacy, in the UK, and in some states in the US, the birth mother is regarded as the legal mother despite her lack of any genetic link to the child. Not only is the Surrogate seen as the legal parent, but if she is married, her husband is regarded as being the other legal parent.

This can be changed by applying for a Parental Order

(see Chapter 8. for more details). In the UK an Order cannot be applied for until after a 'cooling-off' period of six weeks. However, in some US States such as California, an Order can be applied for during the pregnancy. This means that the parental rights of the Intended Parents have been granted before the birth of the baby takes place. In other States, even though the Surrogate is unrelated to the child, the Intended Mother may still be required to adopt the child. The best States are those that allow a Pre-Birth Order, which enables both of the Intended Parents' names to be listed on the birth certificate at birth, and also gives them parental rights immediately after the baby is born.

In some cases, a Gestational Surrogate may decide that she doesn't want to give the baby up. Certainly in the UK, where surrogacy agreements/contracts are not seen as legally binding, clear laws are required that outline what to do in complex situations involving Gestational Surrogacy. Overall, the ability of the law to deal with surrogacy arrangements varies from country to country (and in the case of the US, from State to State). This is discussed further in Chapters 7 and 8.

2. Surrogacy
— Is it for You?

"We were told that we could not have a baby naturally on our own as my uterus was badly scarred after a really bad miscarriage several years ago. I have been trying to get pregnant ever since. I have had five attempts at IVF, and even used a donated egg on the last attempt. Nothing worked for us. We have now, after five years of trying, decided to use a Surrogate. The decision was the hardest and scariest thing we have ever decided as a couple in our entire 15 years of marriage." Neil & Dawn, Sydney, Australia

The best way to make an informed decision about whether surrogacy might be the way forward for you is to find out as much as possible about it first. In this chapter I deal with the most frequently asked questions (FAQs) by Intended Parents. In the remainder of the book you will find further details about the process and, importantly, the legal position in the UK and overseas. If you decide to proceed with a surrogate pregnancy, you will find it invaluable to return to this information along the way. You might also find it helpful to show this book to the family members, friends and professionals who will be involved too.

What should be considered when making a decision for or against surrogacy?

Surrogacy is a last option for many couples. Strict adoption and fostering laws make it impossible for a couple over a certain age to apply for a child through their local authority, or even to adopt outside of their country. Meanwhile same-sex couples are still shunned by the authorities in some parts of the UK, and even in those areas of the country where they are encouraged to apply to adopt or foster, are not always given the welcome that they deserve. These are some of the reasons why so many people have turned to adoption overseas during the years, and why they are now turning to surrogacy as a way forward instead.

The decision at the end of the day has to be reached by you. Only you know your personal circumstances — better than any social worker. Your ability to parent would not come into question if you were able to reproduce yourself 'naturally' (unless of course you had been referred to social services because of something in your past that would put into question your ability to parent). Often, you would become a parent without even consciously choosing to do so beforehand.

In most cases of surrogacy, those who go through the challenges to reach the end point have normally come to terms with the fact that, for them, getting pregnant is not an option. In the process, they have given a great deal more thought to their suitability to parent than the vast majority of other parents. However, surrogacy is inevitably still a difficult journey.

Take into account your support network: what is it like? Who will be there to support you when you are going through the IVF attempts? Who will be there when the IVF isn't successful? — because the reality is that not all IVF cycles work first time around. Who will be there when the baby is born? And what if you have multiples from your first IVF transfer? Will you be able to cope with the extra mouths to feed and the extra care needed to look after them? If you need to work with an Egg Donor, have you come to terms with the fact that one of you will not be the biological parent? And if you are a woman, have you come to terms with the fact that the baby you are about to parent is biologically your partner's, but (in most cases) is not your own?

Once you come to terms with all these questions, you are ready to go.

Is surrogacy just for couples?

The simple answer to this should be NO! You should be able, regardless of your couple status, to access the services of a Surrogate and/or Egg Donor. Unfortunately, however, the laws are different for each country in terms of their acceptance of surrogacy. What they class as legal surrogacy can sometimes disallow a single person from going through surrogacy. This is because applications for Parental Orders may only be open to married couples, or to couples who can show that they were in a committed relationship when the baby was conceived.

What I will say is that single people have been travelling abroad for many years to utilize surrogacy services in countries that are very open to working with them. And throughout the UK, children have been born to single men and women with the help of a Surrogate and Egg Donor. However, while you will be legally recognized as the parent in the USA, the UK does not allow single people to use a Surrogate in terms of applying for a Parental Order.

How does surrogacy work for gay couples and singles?

Gay men and women have been parents for many years. There are thousands of gay parents in the UK now, so many that there is an annual Alternative Families show in London where attendance continues to grow year on year. Most gay parents have had children within heterosexual relationships before the gay parent 'came out', while others have made co-parenting agreements with other gay friends. However, surrogacy for same-sex partners has been around for years too: over 16 years in the US; and 13 years in the UK. The rest of the world are currently playing catch-up, but boy are they catching up fast!

In the UK, my partner and I were the first same-sex couple to use a Surrogate Mother to have children. Our journey to have our Surrogate babies started in 1996/7, and our first set of twins were born in California in the winter of December 1999. We arrived back into the UK in late December, in time to celebrate New Year's Eve with our family and friends. It was the best Christmas and New Year of our lives. Surrogacy for same-sex couples has grown exponentially since then. These days it is not uncommon to walk around San Francisco's Castro area and see numbers of gay single men and couples pushing their babies around. The same is happening all over the globe, from Australia to Germany. The UK is no different; even London Zoo has an annual "Gay Day" where hundreds of gay families travel from all over the country to spend the day with other gay families.

Same-sex singles and couples should note, though, that there are specific State- and country specific laws that are applicable to them when using a Surrogate. California allows same-sex couples to apply for a Pre Birth Order (PBO) from about the fourth month of the pregnancy, while the UK allows same-sex couples to apply for a Parental Order six weeks after the birth of the baby. However, this is not the case everywhere.

Further information about the legal situation for same-sex singles and couples can be found in Chapters 7 & 8. Please ensure you have an agency working with you, or if you are independent from an agency, get proper legal advice. You must safeguard yourself from Day One. There is further information about sources of support in Appendix C.

How does surrogacy work
for people living with disability?

Pretty much the same way as it does for those people living without disability, to be honest. As with all Intending Parents, you must take into account the amount of work and commitment that will be needed to look after any children born through surrogacy. Once you are fully committed to the process and you have organised the support network around you that you will need to do the daily care, go for it!

Your disability should not prevent your being able to get access to the services of a Surrogate Mother, or indeed to an Egg Donor. If being a parent is important enough to you, you will overcome any disability related obstacle in your way. Disabled people make fantastic parents too, and should be given the opportunities which are now available through surrogacy to show that.

What is the emotional impact of using a Surrogate?

I see hundreds of couples and singles every year who are considering surrogacy, and they come in all shapes and sizes and with all sorts of emotional baggage. Your situation, no matter how bad it has been for you, has been gone through a hundred times by other couples before it started to be an issue for you.

The stress of going through years of IVF cycles will have taken its toll on many of you who have been through this process before. I regularly see heterosexual couples who have had years of attempts themselves, with miscarriage after miscarriage and failed cycles after failed cycles. Most are feeling downbeat and apprehensive about the next steps forward, and about what surrogacy can do for them. These couples usually have a very strong relationship by this point, and are ready for the rollercoaster ride that could be still waiting for them. In most cases, the Intended Parents have already supported each other through similar emotional and practical strain for years, and are still ready to go on and be supportive to their partners come what may.

Our same-sex couples are somewhat different in their approach. Over the years, I have seen several long-term partnerships break down because of the surrogacy process. Gay couples normally come into surrogacy as being the ONLY way for them to have a biological child of their own. Some men may have children as a result of a relationship with a woman years beforehand, but a gay male couple cannot have a biological baby together without the help of a Surrogate and an Egg Donor.

With this in mind, gay couples tend to come to us without the experience of IVF clinics or of having to fight through infertility issues. (The benefit of this, of course, is that they have no emotional scarring as a result of past experience of the IVF procedure.) Most, if not all, are at the top of their game professionally, and all are used to a certain level of service from the suppliers that they utilize. Many regard the surrogacy process as a professional service that they are obtaining to help them build their family, and most want to have a professional experience.

As a result of many years of experiencing the gay community accessing surrogacy services, a considerable number of Surrogates across the world will only work with gay couples/singles. These women argue that the relationship between the Surrogate and the Intended male Parents is less intense than it can be between the Intended Mother(s) and Surrogate with a heterosexual or female couple. This is because when a male couple is involved, the experiences that an Intended Mother has gone through with her own infertility over the years is not transferred to the Surrogate during the pregnancy. This transference of feelings and experiences is some-times the cause of much mediation during the preg-nancy, and causes unneeded tension to the Surrogate. (Though as with all negative surrogacy experiences, it can be avoided with careful planning and the right advice and support.)

Whatever your situation, the aim should be for everyone involved to have as emotionally comfortable journey as possible.

What kind of woman volunteers to become a Surrogate?

The majority of Western Surrogates are from lower-middle-class backgrounds. They tend to be housewives or 'stay-at-home moms', or at most have part-time jobs and devote their real energies to parenting.

Most of the women I have met who have chosen to become Surrogates have said the same thing. They have either witnessed infertility in a relative or friend that drew them to want to help, or they have seen friends become Surrogates and thought that they could do something similar. In either case, they recognize their contribution to the process as being a wonderful gift that they are giving to the Intended Parents, helping another family to do something that could not be done otherwise. This is the main guiding force that compels them to become Surrogate Mothers.

Critics of surrogacy will always try to play the "babies

for sale" card, or the "creating designer babies card", but the reality is that the amount of compensation you actually pay your Surrogate would not even cover the minimum wage in most countries for the amount of hours necessary to carry a pregnancy to term. The single characteristic that can be used to describe women who choose to become Surrogates is altruism. In the US and UK, the amount of expenses/financial compensation that each Surrogate gets depends on the experience she has gained in the field, but it is not the primary factor that determines her becoming a Surrogate.

Surrogates are mostly caring compassionate women who have a sense of what a childless couple or single is feeling in not being able to carry a baby themselves, and who really want to help create and be a part of something wonderful. However, saying that, I have met many Surrogates and potential Surrogates over the years who have only thought about the compensation package that they are going to receive. These are the women that you need to weed out and stay away from.

Undesirable Surrogates tend to come with a long list of demands from the start, telling you what it is that they are looking for in terms of financial base fees, home help, childcare and a variety of other extras on top. Some of the demands are outrageous; others are more realistic and are open for discussion. In any case, you should only work with someone who you find ethically sound in terms of their expectations, and who is realistic about what you are going to be able to provide to her once she is pregnant and carrying your baby.

How do I find a Surrogate?

Most Intended Parents seek a 'professional' Surrogate, one who has been through the process in the past and who is clearly looking to help other Intended Parents to create a family. The logic is that she has been through the process at least once before, and therefore knows what is needed from her. She is also more likely to give up the child at the end of the process if she has been able to do it in the past. She knows the protocol that was used during her last surrogacy, and your clinic can request to see these protocols and her medical notes to make sure there were no problems the previous time.

There are country specific requirements that you will need to consider when looking for your Surrogate. In the US, there are actually State laws that set out the legal process you need to follow when using a Surrogate who resides and will deliver the baby in that State. It is crucial that you get proper advice when starting the search, and stay within the law for each country or State you are searching in.

An easy way to find a Surrogate or Egg Donor in the US is to advertise for one — magazines, newspapers and internet forums are the usual places. The British Surrogacy Centre actively flyers university campuses around the US to attract Egg Donors into their programme, and this works extremely well, in California we also have staff members who go into shopping malls and set up stands to attract potential Surrogates to us. The type of Egg Donor you want is down to your choice, of course, but you are more likely to find what it is you are looking for on a university campus then walking around a shopping mall. In terms of your Surrogate, though, the reverse is the case.

However, in the UK and other countries where commercial surrogacy is illegal, advertising for Surrogates is not allowed. In the UK, it is also against the law for a woman to advertise herself as a potential Surrogate under the Surrogacy Act 1985. It is odd that surrogacy itself is NOT illegal, but that advertising is. Despite this, Surrogates based in the UK, and Intended Parents searching for a Surrogate, can advertise on internet boards and newspapers based outside of the UK. Where there's a will, there's a way!

The best way to find a Surrogate if you live in a country where it is illegal to advertise is to go through an agency, or, if you prefer to work independently of an agency, to advertise on message boards based overseas. So long as you find an overseas message board that has an international audience, it might well match you with someone who is geographically local to you.

Can a foreign couple work with a Surrogate in another country?

Each country and State has its own rules about Intended Parents from overseas being able to use Surrogates who are residents there. You will need to research these regulations and make sure that you are not breaking any laws. It is legal, for example, for a Surrogate in California to give birth for a couple (or single) who are resident outside of the US, which is why many couples go there from countries around the world. In the UK, a Surrogate cannot give birth for a couple who are domiciled outside the country.

Once you have identified a Surrogate, what are the checks and tests that need to be done?

As a general rule, a Gestational Surrogate is chosen on the basis of her general health. Many parents like to seek a gestational carrier who has already had at least one child, indicating that she is capable of carrying a baby safely to term. Otherwise, it is advisable to use one of the range of ovulation tests on the market to check that your Surrogate is fertile.

If you are working with the help of facilitators like the British Surrogacy Centre, they will have performed all the necessary police checks that they recommend beforehand. Otherwise, I would strongly advise that you obtain a Criminal Records Bureau (CRB) or country equivalent check for the Surrogate and her husband before going ahead.

A centre like the British Surrogacy Centre will also arrange for testing to be carried out for HIV and other STDs on the Surrogate and the Intended Parents. Otherwise, it is important to check for at least the following: HIV; Chlamydia; Gonorrhoea; Hepatitis B; Hepatitis C; and Syphilis.

It is also advisable for the Intended Father to have a sperm analysis performed, to ascertain that the sperm is of a high enough quality to fertilise an egg without assistance. At this stage, if problems with sperm quality become apparent, the agency can make arrangements to perform ICSI. This is where a single sperm is injected directly into the egg (see Chapter 4. for more details) to help with the fertility process. Otherwise, an IVF treatment cycle will be wasted, which is very costly in terms of money, emotion and time. I recently heard of a facility in the UK that performed ICSI free of charge for certain patients who were going through financial hardship rather than letting them waste that IVF cycle.

What would it cost?

How long is a piece of string? This is the million-dollar question. Nothing if you were lucky enough to win the new To-Hatch IVF Lotto that's just being launched by Camilla Strachan. (Yes, really.) The reality is that surrogacy costs are different everywhere in the world. In the UK, where commercial surrogacy is illegal, the costs run anywhere from £30,000- £70,000. This is dependent on where you go for treatment, and the terms that you reach with your Surrogate (and your Egg Donor if you need one).

Surrogates' legal compensation should be around £12-15,000, but there are pockets of Surrogates springing up around the UK who 'sell' themselves as being altruistic, but who in reality hire themselves out at between £19,000 and £25,000 a time. Not only is this illegal to do, it is unethical. Many of these Surrogates will argue that they deserve the higher amounts because they are 'proven' Surrogates, but they are not horses or breeder cows. The number of times that a woman goes through a surrogacy journey should not mean that she can up her base fee each time. In most cases, these Surrogates come with far too much baggage anyway.

Unethical Surrogates are not normally prepared to work through centres or agencies, under the pretence that they are trying to save the Intended Parents money. The reality is that they want to be able to use the fact that there is no third party to go through as a way to pressure you throughout the pregnancy into parting with more money. I have known Surrogates demand the most ridiculous things once they are pregnant; almost holding their Intended Parents to ransom. The Intended Parents fear to say no, in case the Surrogate takes revenge in some way or another. This is why it is important to ensure that everything is in the contract you set up with the Surrogate (see below, and see Chapter 8 for further legal advice). Make the Surrogate aware that you will honour what's in the contract, but if its NOT in the contract, not to ask for it as refusal often offends.

There are an alarming number of UK-based Surrogates who try to set themselves up as being 'experts' in surrogacy. Some of these women carry a lot of valuable information about the practical side of surrogacy, but they are NOT professionals. They tend to see surrogacy only from the Surrogate's point of view, which can become clouded if they have had a bad experience in the past with their previous Intended Parents. These Surrogates tend to sit on internet forums, spending hours each day waiting for the next bit of gossip that they can get their teeth into. Many Intended Parents have fallen foul of a bitter Surrogate's tongue on these forums, and have found their whole lives revealed to anyone who wants to listen.

I always say to the Intended Parents that I come into contact with, don't be tempted to try and find a Surrogate online. Let the professionals do it for you and vet them for you, so that you don't have to spend the whole pregnancy utilising mediation services because of the breakdown that's occurred because of a bad match. Not every Surrogate is the right Surrogate for you, and just because one Surrogate says she will work for you, don't feel like you have to grab her before she goes and finds another couple. If she is the right Surrogate, she will wait, because she also wants to have a good experience. If you meet a woman who gives you a time limit to get contracts and so on done and says that otherwise she is going to find another couple to work with, then say goodbye: she is the wrong person for you.

In the US, costs average around $90,000-$120,000, but again, it will depend on the clinic that you use and the terms you agree with your Surrogate and Egg Donor. It will also depend on which law firm you work with and, if you are working with an agency or centre, if they have a rate card set up with the lawyers to give you discounts on their services. Every agency and every centre should be recommending a service provider to you who will give you a good price. It is essential that *you* get the benefit of discounts and not them.

Think about it from a business perspective: if legal fees are going to cost you around $12-15,000 on the US side, and if I recommend 30-40 clients per annum to a particular legal firm, then although legally they cannot pay me a commission, they can reduce the rates they charge my referrals to retain my future business. Every agency and centre has the ability to ask for this price reduction, and they should be passing on the cost benefits to you rather than retaining these for themselves.

In the UK, over many years we have seen fees of between £30,000-£50,000 being charged by 'expert' law firms to vulnerable clients who have just returned form overseas with their babies, for help with Parental Orders etc. As the British Surrogacy Centre, we have arranged fixed prices with a couple of UK firms to establish parental rights in the UK for a fraction of this cost. It is important that you ensure you are fully informed about your choices. The options are out there, you just have to look for them. If someone wants to charge you £30,000-£50,000 to sort out your Parental Orders, run a mile!

At the cheapest end, costs in India and the Ukraine range from around £15,000-£40,000, depending on the route you take and if you are willing to use a Surrogate who is housed like a battery hen. The disgraceful conditions that some of these women are kept in is totally immoral, and should not be allowed. Unfortunately, some Intended Parents are just not able to afford the fees that are paid to UK or US-based Surrogates.

How do you ensure that the Surrogate isn't being exploited?

It is important to make sure that the Surrogate you work with is not just doing this for the money that she may earn whilst she is carrying your baby. It is equally important not to work with a Surrogate who is being forced by a partner or 'friend' to be your Surrogate. Only with due diligence will you be able to work out if this is the case or not. Do the checks and ask the questions; if you don't get straight answers, walk away.

In places like India and Thailand, we see women who are forced into surrogacy at the hands of greedy relatives and pimps. These people have worked out that they can make more money in a year keeping 20 girls in a house pregnant, than through shipping clients in and out all day for prostitution services. A Surrogate in India can earn a hundred times the amount of money in a year than most women in India would earn in five years. This is why it is important to be extremely cautious when considering using a Surrogate in countries like these. You also need to be aware that there are clinics opening up in other parts of the world like the US where couples are being sent to India or the Ukraine for the actual surrogacy service.

Many people who condemn all cases of surrogacy feel that it is by its very nature immoral, and exploits women and their families who are living in poverty. Just like other aspects of life that cause controversy, unless you are involved in surrogacy, it can seem hard to understand when you are on the outside looking in. The fact is that, unless you have been in the position yourself of being told you are infertile, or that because of your age or sexual orientation you cannot be considered for adoption or fostering, you can have no idea how people feel who are going through it right now. Similarly, surrogacy critics have no understanding of what motivates Surrogate Mothers beyond money. But just because there are those people who do not understand what you are going through, don't let them spoil it for you. It is just their ignorance that is making them feel the way they do.

One of the roles of the British Surrogacy Centre is to educate people about surrogacy and how it can be conducted ethically. We have classes set up to talk about the issues surrounding surrogacy, and classes for extended family members to take them through the process too and to help them to understand what has gone into creating the Intended Parents' children.

Who can be a Surrogate Mother and does my age exclude me?

Any woman between the ages of 20-42 will make a brilliant Surrogate, as long as their fertility history doesn't show that there are areas of concern. In fact, one of our Surrogate Mothers was 45 when she delivered our last set of twins. We had a very healthy pregnancy and a fantastic delivery. I have known women as old as 53 give birth to babies that were conceived through IVF and donated eggs, and who sailed through the pregnancy. However, there are some doctors in the UK, for example, who will not work with women over 37.

What is the best way to create a good relationship with the Surrogate?

The relationship that a family has with a Surrogate will vary depending on the amount of contact that you want to have with each other. Some Intended Parents want to be as involved as possible in the pregnancy, and this certainly works for a lot of Surrogates. But there are also those Intended Parents who either cannot be that involved because of the distance between their geographical locations, or because they just do not want to be that friendly with their Surrogate. There are also Surrogates who feel that they want to maintain a friendly relationship with their Intended Parents, but no more than that.

In any case, the amount and nature of contact is usually clearly spelled out in a contract agreed to by all parties before the pregnancy commences. However, contracts between you and your Surrogate are not legally binding in some countries. The UK does not recognise a surrogacy contract; California, on the other hand, has a different approach and finds all contracts legally binding. Again, you need to look at country specific guidelines to establish what needs to be done.

I advise you to establish a contract anyway, regardless of where you are living, as it sets out clearly what the intention was throughout the arrangement. This will help you clear up any issues later that your Surrogate brings up. I say if it's NOT in the contract, then it doesn't happen.

During the pregnancy, a Surrogate may be asked to follow certain health guidelines, such as not smoking, drinking, or using drugs. She is also required to attend regular prenatal check-ups, and to observe basic precautions to protect the health of the developing foetus. Depending on the terms agreed in the contract, a gestational carrier may visit or communicate via telephone or email to keep you updated on the pregnancy, or she may maintain minimal contact. It's really up to you.

Will there be an ongoing relationship with the Surrogate?

In most cases a gestational carrier will give up all rights to the resulting child; after all, there is no genetic link between them whatsoever. Some Intending Parents maintain a relationship with their Surrogate for life, though. I personally never went into either of my surrogacy journeys wanting a new best friend, but in both cases I did end up with best friends for life. However, it is not normal for the Surrogate to participate in child-rearing at all. Parents and potential Surrogates should think about these issues carefully before making an agreement, and they should take the time to discuss expectations before deciding on going forward together.

Are solicitors really needed or just an unnecessary waste of money?

In my opinion, you must have a lawyer to represent your interests. But as in any industry, there are good ones and bad ones, expensive ones and less expensive ones, and those with surrogacy experience and those without. Don't assume that, just because someone shouts the loudest on a subject — even if they have convinced a newspaper to run with the headline that they are the industry expert — that they know what they are doing. Look at their credentials and check these carefully. Remember, this area of law has not been around for long, and real experts are not made overnight! Being an expert comes with time and expe-rience of working on many surrogacy cases.

At the British Surrogacy Centre, we hear stories all the time about people who have ended up with £30,000-£50,000 bills from firms in the City of London. They have almost scared clients to death with stories of children being sent out of the country or refused entry to the UK because they have resulted from a Surrogate births. This is not correct. We have never heard of a baby who has been refused entry into the UK once it has arrived from abroad.

In fact, the opposite is the case. The immigration officials in the UK have been, to date, quite accommodating with couples and singles coming back to the UK with their baby or babies. There is a legal process that immigration officials must go through with you, and they will give you a step-by-step account of what you need to do next in order for your baby to remain in the country with you. At this point, you must follow the guidelines and make the necessary arrangements in conjunction with your solicitor.

It is vitally important that you do the things you need to do as soon as you can, because if the immigration service have given you a fixed amount of time to get the paperwork lodged with them, you need to adhere to this timeframe so that the child can legally stay. It is not worth taking the risk that your child will be asked to leave. You will find that the UK immigration service is actually a very reasonable body to work with. There are lots of misconceptions floating around about how you will be treated by them, but it has been my experience that they have been extremely compassionate and accommodating to all of the families that we have helped over many years.

Apart from contracts before the birth and immigration and custody arrangements afterwards, as soon as you know that your Surrogate is pregnant, you need to think about changing your Will. It is important to ensure that, if anything should happen to you during the pregnancy, you have put things in place for someone to take your baby at birth and that the Surrogate and baby are taken care of financially. Again, it is best to do this with a solicitor who already has experience of surrogacy arrangements, although your own family law firm will be able to assist you with changing your Will.

How do we ensure that the baby is legally ours?

Chapter 8. covers the legal process in detail, and has been written in conjunction with one of the UK's leading solicitors working in the area of surrogacy. It is important to remember that, if you use a Surrogate overseas, you will need to comply with the UK law as well as the law that applies in the country where she is based. You will need to have a law firm representing you in the country where the Surrogate is based, and another in your own country.

What happens if the foetus or baby is disabled?

All surrogacy contracts, whether legally binding in your country or not, should be used as a tool to show what medical procedures you will expect your Surrogate to undergo while she is carrying your baby. These include tests for indicators of genetic and physical disabilities that some parents would not want to live with (for whatever reason) once the baby is born. It is important to know your capabilities, and to identify what your expectations of your Surrogate would be if you were faced with having a possibly disabled child.

What I mean by this is simple, would you be prepared to care for a child that had any form of disability, or would you not be able to cope? If you do not think that you would be able to cope and that you would expect your Surrogate to have an abortion, then it is important from the beginning of the selection process to be clear that the Surrogate is okay with going through those procedures. It might be that you have a religious Surrogate who does not believe in abortion, and she will not go through with one even if the child has little chance of surviving the birth.

Personally, although I would never have wished to have had a disabled child and all the discomfort and issues it would have brought to one of my children, I would not have been able to terminate the pregnancy. However, I have counseled many couples who have been through the surrogacy journey, and who have terminated a pregnancy because they have felt that they would not have given 100% to the child if it had been born. It is not a nice experience or decision to make, but bear in mind that it may well happen.

You also need to remember that, as with any pregnancy, a baby may become disabled as a result of birth trauma or prematurity, or may be carrying problems that no medical test can predict; no child comes with guarantees. Many children also become disabled as a result of accidents or illnesses in early childhood. If you are absolutely clear that you could not deal with difficulties of any kind, then you should not be considering becoming a parent.

What is the best way to tell family and friends about our plans?

You know your family and friends better than I do. Some will open the champagne and want to celebrate there and then with you, others will show no emotion whatsoever or will be negative, but real friends and loving family members will stand by you no matter what. Be honest and upfront about your surrogacy only when you are ready to do so.

Don't feel that you have to rush to tell everyone; perhaps have just one or two friends who you tell initially. Some people only tell their family and friends once they are expecting their baby, as they previously went through so much trying to get pregnant themselves. Whatever your decision, it's up to you when you tell people and how you tell people.

Would there be problems bonding with the baby?

Over the years I've seen people react to the arrival of their baby in lots of different ways. Those Intended Parents who have been actively involved with their Surrogate during the pregnancy tend to be much more responsive to the baby when it's born, but not in all cases. I've also seen Intended Parents who have had little to do with the pregnancy because of work and geographical location, but who have bonded straight-away. I don't think anyone has denied the bonding sensation of holding your baby for the first time, even if you didn't carry it yourself. The overwhelming love you feel and the unconditional love coming back from your baby will help the bonding process no end!

Fathers tend to bond more quickly with the babies, in my experience, than mothers do. This could well be the fatherly bond that results from birth of every man's child, because he has never physically carried the baby himself. Whereas the Intended Mother would have normally spent the past nine months touching and feeling her growing baby, and would have spent some of that time talking to her bump. Not having experienced this part of the process can sometimes leave the Intended Mother feeling left out, but this quickly goes away. She is soon smitten with her new bundle of joy, and her own maternal feelings soon show themselves.

Depending on which agency you are working with, they will have offered counseling throughout the process for you anyway. This would be a great time to discuss any concerns you have, and to find ways to work through any issues that might show itself. Don't be afraid to ask for help.

What is the best way to tell the children about their origins?

Over the years this question has come up hundreds of times. The simple answer is that you have to judge yourself when the time is right to tell your child or children about its origins. In the case of a Sperm Donor, most countries have laws that will make certain information available to children born through sperm donation when they reach 18, so it is important to disclose this to them yourself. In terms of surrogacy, what you tell your child will depend on the circumstances of the case. For example, if your baby was born with the help of the Surrogate and an Egg Donor, there are lots of issues to consider. Not only the birth, but also the biological miss-link. However, it might be that if you were able to use your own egg and partner's sperm; then the only thing you might want to talk to the child about is that another lady helped you start your family.

Some parents and Surrogates will have lifelong friendships; others will have nothing to do with each other at all at the end of the process. Now that birth certificates are able to bear the names of the Intended Parents and not those of the Surrogate or the Egg Donor, some parents will not tell their children anything. Certainly in countries like France and Germany, where surrogacy is illegal, the child will be passed off as the child of the Intended Parents through-out its life. However, adult children of Sperm Donors advocate strongly for the importance of disclosure.

Personally, we have been up-front with our children from a very early age. They are aware that we had an Egg Donor, and that we used the help of a Surrogate Mother to carry them to term. They know each of the women personally, and talk with them on a regular basis. Each of the women involved have promised to be there in later life to answer any questions the children will have, and this works really well for us. Our children know who their parents are, and who else was involved in the process of their birth.

Are there any other parenting issues to consider?

A child born through surrogacy does not need to be parented any differently to a child born the 'traditional' way. However, parents may face different issues. There may be eyebrows raised at the school when one of the parents waiting for pick-ups or drop-offs is a little older than the other parents in the playground, or when the mother uses a wheelchair, but this would always be the case. If it is known that a woman can still produce eggs from her intact ovaries, but couldn't carry her child herself and had the assistance of another woman for that part of the process, though, then eyebrows will certainly be raised. Similarly two men — or two women — waiting at the playground gates will obviously have had help to have their family.

Over the next ten years, educators and hospital staff to name but a few will have to deal with a whole new family system coming through their front doors. Training these professionals will have to include training about the structure of the families utilizing their services. Professionals will have to cope with not only their own views towards surrogacy, and indeed towards same-sex parenting, but also with the attitudes of other parents at the school or patients within the hospital which may not be as tolerant.

There are those people who will go out of their way to make sure that your children are treated no differently than their peers. Then there are those who just stay away, but worst of all are those who show the world that they are treating them no differently to others by going over the top, overtly treating the children in a way that could be seen discriminatory.

43

Over the years, I have seen both sides of the fence. I have had to go into the school office after complaints from other parents about my showing affection to my partner in the school playground (this apparently being inappropriate for other children to see). I have had to advocate for my children not wanting to make a Mother's Day card with the rest of the class, but wanting to make one for Grandma instead (again, this is not a situation unique to families who have used surrogacy). I have also had to deal with my children not getting the invites to the class parties that others have had. However, we have survived it all, and are stronger as a family as a result.

Is there further support available, both now and in the future?

Appendix C provides details of agencies, solicitors, internet sites and other sources of support and information. The British Surrogacy Centre runs parenting skills evenings, and holds monthly groups for heterosexual and same-sex parents. The aim is to confront issues that may arise, and to get other peoples' views on their own experiences and to talk through possible scenarios of what may come up with professionals from all walks of life.

3. 10 Steps to Parenthood via Surrogacy

"The best thing that we ever did was to find a Surrogate and Egg Donor to complete our family — we are now a 'proper' family!"
Jason and Paul, London, UK

This chapter concentrates on Gestational Surrogacy: however, the same principles apply apart from the use of the clinicians. Most Traditional Surrogacy is carried out with Home Insemination, which is explained in the following chapter.

Step 1: Find the right help

Once you have decided that surrogacy is for you, you need to decide if you are going to be able to facilitate the surrogacy yourself, or whether you should bring in an agency or facilitator to organise things for you. Deciding which way to go will largely depend on your own ability to pull everything together for the surrogacy, and where in the world you live. Many couples decide that, for their first surrogacy at least, they will get professional help.

There are agencies all around the world that can help you with your surrogacy. Some are better than others, and some have higher success rates at providing a 'happy ending' than others. It is best to be cautious when looking at reviews online. Some agencies have been around for many successful years and have still had minor setbacks with Surrogates or Intending Parents, while positive reviews of other agencies may hide underlying problems. Not everyone is happy with everything, and ultimately you can only judge an agency by how they treat you.

Once you have decided which facilitator to use, you should arrange an introductory consultation to talk about your needs. There are companies all over the world that will want to charge for your initial consultation with them; don't touch these with a bargepole. At the end of the day, if they want your business — and make no mistake, it is a multi-million-pound a year business — they should be meeting with you for no charge and selling themselves to you.

At this initial meeting, the facilitator will discuss all the options available to you. You should be advised on every aspect of surrogacy, and be given the opportunity to ask questions. If you choose an out-of-town or international agency to work with, you may well have to fly over to meet them. However, lots of agencies will work online with you, and some even tour regions, holding meetings in hotels and other venues.

However you make your initial contact with an

agency, ask them the following questions:

i. How long have you been in business and where are your offices?
ii. How many couples are you currently working with?
iii. How many couples have you helped in the past?
iv. Which fertility clinics do you work with?
v. What's the waiting time for a Surrogate to be found?
vi. What's the waiting time for an Egg Donor to be found?
vii. What's the cost?
viii. How are your Surrogates and Egg Donors vetted?
ix. Is there a money-back option if the Surrogate does not get pregnant?
x. Will you give discounts after the first failed transfer and thereafter?
xi. What on-going support do you give e.g. with birth certificates/ passports?
xii. What do they know about the laws in your country; do they have a representative in your country to help you if needed?

and then anything else you can think of yourselves.

Step 2: Sign the agency contract

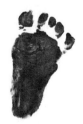

After the initial meeting, the contracts and particularly the Retainer agreement need to be discussed. When you are sure that surrogacy is for you and that you are happy to work with the agency, you will be given the

Retainer agreement to sign. At this point your surrogacy becomes real, and the agency will work with you to find you the perfect Surrogate and/or Egg Donor. Please be prepared to wait, though, for a good Surrogate to become available. Do not rush into signing a contract with the first one who offers because you feel that you just want to get the process underway. The best ones really are worth waiting for!

Step 3:
Register with a clinic

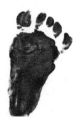

The clinic is where egg donation and embryo transfer will take place. It is crucial that all parties to the surrogacy have medical screening beforehand, so registration with a clinic is the next step. If you are local to your clinic, you would enrol with their programme and meet them in person. If you are travelling from another country or from out of the area, then you would have a telephone enrolment via a three-way telephone call between you, the agency and the clinician.

All medical testing will need to be performed to country specific guidelines. Depending on which clinic you decide to work with, they might have their own requirements on the tests they want you to undergo, but all clinics will require at least HIV and other STD testing. Most will also require you to undergo counseling and psychotherapy sessions, but not all. It is recommended that you also have any sperm that is going to be used tested and frozen at this time to help to cut down waiting times later.

Step 4: Search for the right Egg Donor and Surrogate Mother

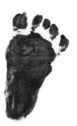

Your facilitator will be using the time that you are waiting for the quarantine period to end for the sperm to match you up with your Surrogate, and if needed, with an Egg Donor too. Finding the perfect Surrogate is a difficult job. You have to let the facilitator know what type of Surrogate you are looking to work with. You need to be upfront about the type of relationship that you are looking for, whether that be an involved, hands-on approach, or more of a closed relationship where you might just go through the surrogacy talking every now and again with the Surrogate following medical appointments etc.

It is important to remember that no agency in the world has a waiting list of Surrogates and Egg Donors. If you are told that this is the case, they are not the right agency to work with. Rather, most agencies are really busy on Mondays and Tuesdays, with emails from potential Surrogates coming in after the previous weekend. This is because lots of potential Surrogates, bored at home, have spent time during the weekend on the internet and have come across the agency's website. Not all of these women turn out to be viable Surrogates, for whatever reason, but, just occasionally, some are perfect.

In order to find your perfect match, you will be asked by the facilitator to create a full biographical profile about you and your partner, and this will need to be completed as soon as possible. Once you have filled out all the profile paperwork, this can be matched with initial possible Egg Donors and Surrogates. You will also provide photos of yourself and partner, and these will form part of your profile assessment that will be shared with the Surrogate and Egg Donor. Names can be left out of the profile if you so wish, but this depends on you and the type of relationship you wish to have with your Surrogate and/or Egg Donor.

Step 5: Finalise your choice of Egg Donor and Surrogate

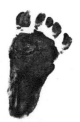

From the database of potential Egg donors and possible Surrogates, the facilitator will select several matches for you. Ultimately, the decision is yours for the choice of Egg Donor, but they should decide a match for you in regards to a suitable Surrogate.

Meeting Surrogates/Egg Donors is completely up to you. Once the facilitator has found several Egg Donor profiles for you to go through and recommended a couple of potential Surrogates, you need to decide if you would like to meet any of them, perhaps at the time when you attend the clinic for testing. If you wish to have an anonymous Egg Donor, this is possible, because the facilitator can give the Egg Donor a number and refer to you only by the first letter of your Christian name.

Step 6: Draw up and sign the contract

Once you have decided on which two wonderful women are going to help you to grow your family, you need to start thinking about contracts for them. This is something that you need to think about very carefully indeed. Some countries have fixed rules on contracts for surrogacy, while in other cases these are not seen as being enforceable documents in a court of law.

In the UK, for example, if you tried to uphold any part of a surrogacy agreement in the courts, the courts would not take anything in the contract into account. In California, though, everything in a surrogacy contract is deemed by the courts to be legally enforceable. As such, if the contract is broken by anyone named in the contract, the courts would get to decide the outcome by taking all reasonable measures to make sure that the contract was upheld.

It is important when putting your contracts together that you have a section in there that mentions what you would like to have happen in the eventuality that the Intended Parents were to die during the pregnancy. You will need to decide who would be the next of kin, and what you would like to see happen to the child/ren if this was the case. This is also a good time to think about updating your wills. At the British Surrogacy Centre, all contracts for Intended Parents show an element of this, and we insist that couples name who will be responsible for their babies if they were to die during the pregnancy.

Step 7: Fertility treatment

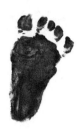

At this stage the physicians will meet with your Surrogate and Egg Donor and ascertain where they are in their menstrual cycle. Each will be put on drugs, and will be monitored over the next few weeks to ascertain when they will be ready for the egg retrieval and later the transfer of embryos. Once this has been determined, the egg retrieval and embryo transfer date will be set. (See Chapter. 5 for the details of how this works.)

Most physicians will want to transfer fresh rather than frozen embryos for the first time at least, so the Surrogate will have been on drugs to regulate her cycle to that of the Egg Donor's to make sure that her uterus is ready for the transfer date. This is normally anywhere between 3-5 days after the retrieval of the eggs.

Once the embryologist has done their bit and has grown the best embryos they can with the material they have, these will be transferred into the Surrogate. Most physicians will not transfer any more than two embryos, because of the excellent success rates of most clinics in achieving a viable pregnancy — most with twins! Our advice to you is by all means increase your chances with the transfer of two embryos, but not any more than two. Transferring three or more embryos will increase the chances of a problematic pregnancy and health problems for the resulting babies.

Now the wait begins!

Step 8: Confirm the pregnancy

At this stage we are looking for a confirmation of pregnancy. A pregnancy test can be done after the 10th day. Be aware that your Surrogate will most definitely have been testing on pee sticks for the past week and not told you about it! The hope is, though, that there is a positive result and you can sit back now and enjoy the pregnancy.

Step 9: Legalise your parenthood

This next, very important step needs to be ongoing throughout your pregnancy. Depending on which country your Surrogate is going to give birth in, you will have to follow a different procedure. The procedure in the UK for gaining Parental Rights is set down by the Government, and you cannot apply until six weeks after the birth. This is seen as the Surrogate's 'cooling off period', where she might change her mind. Even if the baby has no biological link to the Surrogate, she is regarded as being the legal mother and thus has all the rights associated with giving birth to her own child.

In the US, each State is different. California, for example, allows you to establish parental rights to an unborn child. This means that, four months into the pregnancy, the Intending Parents can petition the courts to establish themselves as the legal parents of any children born to the Surrogate between any two given dates. This will also allow you to have your names placed on the original birth certificate at the hospital when the baby is born. In these circumstances, you should aim to establish your parental responsibilities during the first semester.

Step 10: The birth and beyond

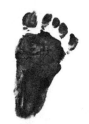

Now for the birth. From the moment your baby is born, s/he becomes your responsibility and you will be expected to look after them. Again, depending on the country where your Surrogate gives birth and the clinic's views on surrogacy, you may need to do certain things. In the US, for example, you will need to show a copy of the Pre-Birth Order to the social work department in the hospital where the birth takes place. This makes them fully aware of the situation, and protocols can be put in place for your baby to come straight to you after the birth.

If your baby is born abroad and the baby is with you, you will need to start chasing up the actual paper copy of the birth certificate. Once you have this, you will need to arrange an appointment at the Passport Office nearest to where you are staying. When your passport has arrived, you are set to leave for home. Please check with your airline about what age they will allow an infant to fly with them.

4. Getting Pregnant via Insemination (Traditional Surrogacy)

The success rate for insemination is the same as with intercourse, perhaps slightly higher as you are being much more precise with timings etc. If you are using frozen semen, you may well have several samples that you can use over a few days, which will help. If you are using donated semen, it is crucial that all proper testing has been carried out beforehand on the donor to eliminate the chances of passing on any STDs. I also recommend that genetic testing is performed as routine.

Where possible, timing for this kind of insemination is the same as for intercourse, and ideally it should be repeated several times during the fertile period. The best time is the day before LH surge (as detected with an ovulation predictor kit); the day of LH surge itself; and the following two-three days (the last day or two being insurance). If you don't have all those options, the day of the LH surge and the day after are best. For further information about how to promote and detect ovulation, see the final section in this chapter.

The chance of getting pregnant by artificial insemination is increased if the Surrogate has healthy fallopian tubes and ovulates regularly. The chances of conceptions are also linked to age. Female fertility decreases after the age of 30, until it is almost zero by the age of 45. For 90% of couples, if treatment is successful, it occurs within the first six cycles of treatment. If conception does not occur by this point, other forms of fertility treatment may be indicated. This may include In Vitro Fertilisation (IVF) and Gamete Intra-Fallopian Transfer (GIFT).

Artificial insemination can also be performed in a stimulated menstrual cycle, where hormone drugs are used to stimulate the ovaries to release an egg. Sometimes this is combined with the woman's natural cycle to increase the chance of conception. This is normally used when several attempts at the natural method of insemination has not worked. The drawback here is that stimulation of the ovaries can lead to multiple eggs being released, and so multiple births are common with this method.

There are some clinics around Europe that offer artificial insemination treatment using donor sperm to single women and lesbian couples. However, at present UK clinics are required to consider the 'need of a child to have a father figure' under a clause in the Human Fertilisation and Embryology Act of 1990. This does not mean that the clinics will not treat you: in fact, most will. Please refer to Appendix C for a list of possible clinics.

Procedure for Home Inseminations

The procedure used for home inseminations of your Surrogate has been used for many years by lesbian couples to start their families. The advantage to this method is that you don't need any fitted equipment, and it is possible for the Surrogate to control the process herself. (Overall, a Traditional Surrogate plays a much more active role within the conception than a Gestational surrogate.) You don't even need a speculum (although you can use one). There are basically three ways of doing an at-home insemination:

1. The so-called Turkey Baster Method. (We have known many couples over the years use an actual turkey baster to get pregnant, but we feel it is at least as effective to use a needleless syringe or an oral medicine syringe.)

2. Insemination using a Cervical Cap, Diaphragm or Instead Cup.

3. Using a Cervical Cap with Access Tube, such as the Oligiosperma Cup from Milex (this needs to be purchased via a doctor). This is a cervical cap with a tube for adding sperm after the cup is in place.

Method 1: Turkey baster (syringe)

You will need:

i. Needleless syringe or oral medicine syringe.

ii. Collection cup (not a condom, as most have spermicide coatings which kill the sperm).
iii. Physiological saline without additives or preservatives.
iv. Tube to attach to syringe (optional).
v. Mild germicidal soap.

You can ask your doctor for a needleless syringe, or you can buy an oral medicine syringe at just about any pharmacist. One that is around four inches long or longer is best. Buy the syringe with a plunger, not a bulb end. Packs are also available from the British Surrogacy Centre (www.Britishsurrogacycentre.com). Both types of syringe work pretty much the same way, but the oral medicine syringes have about a half-inch narrow tip on the end. You can attach a catheter (thin tube) to either type of syringe, but you don't need to and it may waste more of the semen to use one.

Once you have everything you will need, you can begin the process:

i. Take a clean (preferably sterile) glass or plastic cup and have the man ejaculate into it. You can mix in a small amount of physiological saline (without additives/preservatives) to help to get as much sperm as possible into the syringe, but don't need to worry too much about leaving a little behind. NB: If you are using frozen sperm, you need to ask the sperm bank for directions on thawing.

ii. Draw back on the syringe once with nothing but air, then push the air out again.

iii. Draw back on the syringe again, but this time put the end of it into the semen — the vacuum created by pulling back on the stopper will draw the semen into the syringe.

iv. Try to tap out any air bubbles, since you don't want to inject air into your vagina. You can do this by slowly rotating the syringe until the opening is facing up. Tap the air bubbles to the top and then push the plunger in just a small amount, enough to get rid of air without squirting semen out too.

v. Get yourself into a position where you can either stay comfortably for a half hour, or can get into position with only minimal movement. The ideal position is either to have the hips raised, or to lay on your side making sure your pelvis is canted. (Usually the hips provide a natural angle if they are wider than your waist, but if your bed, or whatever you are lying on, is soft, you may want to put a pillow or two underneath your hip.)

vi. Slowly glide the syringe or tube into the vagina until it is close to the cervix — but do not try to get it into the cervix, and do this gently. Your goal is to coat the outside of the cervix with semen, and to deposit as much semen as possible as close to the cervix as you can get it.

vii. Slowly release the semen. If you do it too fast, it will squirt out of the vagina, or at least spray away from the cervix.

viii. If you are concerned about wastage in the syringe, you can use some physiological saline (without additives). You should add some to the syringe, shake it a bit, get the air out, and inject. This is not strictly necessary, since there probably won't be enough wastage to be of any real concern.

ix. Try to have an orgasm. Some experts suggest that using a vibrator for clitoral stimulation produces a bigger, more powerful orgasm, but use whatever method works best for you. The orgasm helps the cervix dip into the vaginal pool and suck up sperm. It helps get more sperm up there, and may speed sperm travel too. Avoid penetration (as in intercourse or with a vibrator), since this will disperse the semen and can knock it off its course.

x. You can use water and mild germicidal soap to clean your supplies if they will have time to dry completely before re-use, or run very hot water over them. Otherwise you can use the physiological saline to clean everything.

Method 2: Cervical Cap

You will need:

i. Cervical cap or 'diaphragm' or Instead cup.
ii. Collection cup.
iii. Needleless syringe or oral medicine syringe.
iv. Physiological saline without additives or preservatives.
v. Mild germicidal soap.

A cervical cap or 'diaphragm' is an item that you are usually fitted with by a doctor for reasons of contraception (!). However, the Instead cup is actually a cup that women use to hold their period blood instead of a tampon or pad, and is available over the counter. Both come with directions on insertion. NB: You may want to practice the procedure beforehand to minimize the risk of spilling the semen.

The process is as follows:

i. You can either have the sperm provider ejaculate directly into the cap/diaphragm/cup, or into another clean receptacle such as a glass or plastic beaker (in which case use the syringe to get the semen from the collection receptacle to the cap/diaphragm/cup).

ii. Fold the cap/diaphragm/cup in half so that the upper rim is closed enough to hold in the semen.

iii. Get into a comfortable position for insertion. Usually, standing with one leg up on a chair/toilet, or sitting wide-legged on a toilet works well.

iv. Once the cap/diaphragm/cup is in place, try to have an orgasm, but avoid penetration. As I mentioned above, some suggest that using a vibrator for clitoral stimulation produces a bigger, more powerful orgasm. The orgasm helps the cervix dip into the vaginal pool and suck up sperm. The aim is to get as much semen up by the cervix as possible, and it should speed sperm travel.

v. Leave the cap/diaphragm/cup in place for at least 2-3 hours, but not more than 12 hours (check directions).

vi. You can use water and a mild germicidal soap to

clean your supplies if they will have time to dry completely before re-use, or run very hot water over them. Otherwise you can use physiological saline to clean everything.

The biggest advantage to this method is that you can move around immediately, since the sperm is held in place next to the cervix and stays there until it travels or until you remove the cap/diaphragm/cup. The only disadvantage is that you need to be fitted for the cervical cap or diaphragm (but not for the Instead cup).

Method 3: Cervical Cap with Tube

You will need:

i. Cervical Cap with Tube.
ii. Collection cup, baggy or condom.
iii. Needleless syringe or oral medicine syringe.
iv. Physiological saline without additives or preservatives.
v. Mild germicidal soap.

This would be basically the same as the cervical cap method discussed above, only you inject the sperm through a tube after the cup is in place. The best device we have found so far is sold by Milex to doctors and medical suppliers. You may need to get it from your doctor, but try the company web site first. The success rate is with this method is also quite high.

Intra-Cervical Insemination (ICSI)

ICSI is one of the more commonly used types of artificial insemination with Traditional Surrogates, and is proving increasingly popular for lesbian couples around the world. It is a painless and quick procedure that helps to deposit the sperm sample directly into the cervix. This can help to increase the chances that sperm will swim through your uterus and fertilize an egg. Couples often opt for ICSI because it is associated with good success rates, and is less expensive than other similar procedures. ICSI is typically performed by a reproductive specialist at your local fertility clinic.

In addition to use within surrogacy, ICSI is of particular benefit to couples facing specific problems with conception. Couples who choose to undergo ICSI are typically fertile and have no underlying problems with their reproductive organs. Couples often choose ICSI when the male partner is having difficulty ejaculating during sexual intercourse, as the procedure allows the sperm to be placed inside the woman artificially. Insemination for infertile couples is successful in 10-40% of cases. Successful treatment often depends on what the cause of infertility was. Conception is more likely to occur when the female partner's natural cycle is combined with hormone treatment to stimulate egg release, although this does carry the associated risk of multiple pregnancies.

The ICSI procedure is relatively straightforward, and can be performed in less than ten minutes. It is typically performed by the reproductive endocrinologist or another health care provider at your local clinic.

The process is as follows:

i. You will be asked to lie down on an examination table. The doctor will insert a speculum into your vagina. This is a plastic or metal instrument that helps to hold open your vagina and expose your cervix.

ii. A thin plastic tube called a catheter is then inserted into your vagina until it reaches your cervix.

iii. Once there, the syringe filled with your donor's (or partner's) sperm is attached to the end of the catheter. The sperm sample is pushed out of the syringe and travels through the catheter, where it is deposited around the cervix.

iv. A soft sponge cap may be placed over your cervix in order to prevent leakage of any sperm. This sponge can be removed between six and eight hours after the procedure.

v. You will be asked to rest for a short time after the procedure has been performed — typically, 30 minutes or so. We would recommend an hour of bed rest, and as with all inseminations we recommend only light housework for the next couple of days and no strenuous activity.

ISCI

Ovulation is the key to a successful pregnancy

A woman is usually able to get pregnant for about five days each month, when ovulation occurs. Ovulation is when an egg is released during the menstrual cycle. This is the woman's most fertile time of the month. It usually occurs 12-16 days before the start of her period, and is easier to detect if her periods are regular. Artificial insemination should only be carried out when the woman is most likely to ovulate. However, because sperm can live for three to five days in a woman's reproductive tract, it is possible to become pregnant if intercourse or insemination occurs several days before ovulation.

Some women find it easy to get pregnant, others don't, but the crucial factor in becoming pregnant is determining when ovulation will occur. If you get it wrong, then you have wasted your time. There is no point in going through any of the procedures above if you cannot pinpoint the day of ovulation. If you do it two or three days before or after the event, you will have missed the opportunity to get pregnant.

A woman's menstrual cycle begins with the first day that her period starts, and ends the day before her next period starts. Ovulation can be detected by a half-degree drop in body temperature, and a change in vaginal discharge. However, blood or urine hormone tests, or ultrasound scans, are usually carried out to calculate accurately the most suitable time for insemination. This improves the chance of the treatment leading to conception. There are various methods to determine the time of ovulation:

i. You could just count the days of your menstrual cycle, although this method is often not very reliable. Ovulation generally occurs on day 14 if your cycle is 28 days long.

ii. Using physical signs such as basal body temperature, cervical position and cervical mucus changes (see below for details). The body temperature chart is a daily recording of body temperature, which is an indicator of ovulation (body temperature will rise after ovulation), but you will need to purchase a high accuracy thermometer.

iii. After menstruation, the cervix undergoes a series of changes in position and texture. During most of the menstrual cycle, the cervix remains firm, like the tip of the nose, and is positioned low and closed. However, as a woman approaches ovulation, the cervix becomes softer, and rises and opens in response to the high levels of oestrogen present at ovulation. These changes, with the production of fertile types of cervical mucus, support the survival and movement of sperm. You can examine your cervix by inserting a clean finger into your vagina. Cervical mucus monitoring involves examining the mucus that is secreted from the cervix, which enables a woman to tell where she is in her cycle and thereby predict the time of ovulation.

iv. Using an ovulation test to predict when you are about to ovulate. When ovulation is about to occur a hormone is released which is called the Luteinizing hormone (LH) surge, and can be detected using an ovulation test. When the test is positive, ovulation will occur over the next 24 to 36 hours.

We recommend that you use any one of the available ovulation test kits available from your local pharmacy.

Stages of Cervical Fluid: Post Menses (after Period)

Stage 1: Lasting 2-3 days CM (cervical mucus) is sticky.
Stage 2: Lasting 2-4 days: CM is creamy or milky — beginning of your Fertile period.
Stage 3: Lasting 1-5 days: Egg White Cervical Mucus (EWCM) — very fertile!
Stage 4: Dry, moist or sticky (infertile)

Peak fertile cervical mucus is thin and stretchy. The cervical mucus will look and have the consistency of egg whites. It is slippery to the touch, and if pulled between the fingertips will stretch 1-10 inches. The colour can be clear or iridescent, and it is extremely wet.

After ovulation, progesterone abruptly suppresses the peak mucus, and the mucus pattern continues with sticky mucus for a day or two and then returns to dryness.

Typically, women in their mid-twenties have EWCM for approximately five days, and for only one-two days by their mid-thirties, but this is not the rule. Many women have several days of EWCM late into their thirties.

If your CM has an unusual odour, consult your GP; this may be a sign of infection. If your CM has the consistency of cottage cheese, this may be a sign of a yeast infection, also consult your GP.

Increasing Cervical Mucus

- Cut back on caffeine and don't smoke!

- Drink at least ten 6oz glasses of water a day.

- Take Evening Primrose Oil: 1,000 IU per day should be taken from Cycle Day 1 to Ovulation.

- Take Flax Seed Oil: 2,000 mg per day should be taken from Ovulation to fertilization.

- Take 1000 mg of Red Raspberry daily: start anytime in the cycle.

- Drink grapefruit juice.

- Take 200mg of Guaifenesin daily from day 5 to day 10 of your menstrual cycle (only use 100% Guaifenesin as other ingredients could have the opposite effect).

Other Ways to Boost Fertility

If you've been trying to conceive without success, making some simple lifestyle changes may increase your chance of conception and help to ensure a healthy pregnancy. However, there are some factors, such as age, ovulation problems, sperm disorders and damaged fallopian tubes, which you can't change, and where possible Intended Parents and Surrogates should screen for these before beginning the process.

• Eat well: if you're a woman, a nutritious, balanced diet will help to improve your general health and well-being, and ensure your body is able to nourish a baby. If you're a man, healthy eating is also important for sperm production. Choose a varied diet containing fresh fruit and vegetables, bread, potatoes, rice and other cereals (wholegrain, where possible), low-fat milk and dairy products, lean meat, fish and other sources of protein.

• Watch your weight: being overweight or very underweight can disrupt periods and hinder conception. A woman with a body mass index (BMI) of more than 29 or less than 19 may find it more difficult to conceive. To work out your BMI, divide your weight in kilograms by your height in metres squared (your height in metres multiplied by itself).

• Drink wisely: women trying to conceive should avoid alcohol completely. Men shouldn't drink more than three or four units a day and should avoid binge drinking to prevent damage to sperm.

• Stop smoking: smoking has been linked to infertility and early menopause in women

The Ultimate Guide to Surrogacy & Home Insemination

and to sperm problems in men. It also reduces the success of fertility treatments.

• Be active: regular moderate exercise (such as brisk walking) for at least 30 minutes a day will help to keep you fit for conception and help to control your weight.

• Keep cool: for optimum sperm production, the testicles need to be a couple of degrees cooler than the rest of the body.

• Avoid tight underwear and jeans, and excessively hot baths and saunas.

• Think about your job: occupations that involve sitting for long periods, such as long-distance lorry driving, or exposure to environmental chemicals such as paints or pesticides, may affect sperm quality. If this is an issue, discuss it with your work supervisor.

Concentrate on your diet

Foods to look out for

A diet which is high in fresh, organic fruit, vegetables and grains is the best kind of diet. Here are some fertility super-foods which women should include in their pre-conceptual diet:

• Citrus fruit — they have a high vitamin C content which has been shown to improve fertility levels.

• Sunflower seeds and nuts for the zinc content.

• Brown rice, oat, pulses and green vegetables for B vitamins. Vitamin B6 is particularly important as it helps to metabolise hormones like oestrogen, which could assist you in getting pregnant. B6 is also good for pregnant women as it breaks down hormones that cause morning sickness, so having plenty of vitamin B6 in the diet can prevent or lessen morning sickness.

• Oily fish for Omega 3, or if you are a vegetarian, linseed or flaxseeds on your breakfast cereal.

Also drink plenty of water, and substitute herb or fruit teas for coffee.

Foods to avoid

There are some fertility killing foods that you should avoid. These are:

• Alcohol — this inhibits your vitamin absorption and can even make you anaemic.

• Tea, coffee and chocolate — these all contain caffeine which also inhibit your body's ability to absorb vitamins. Too much caffeine has also been linked to miscarriage.

• White bread — this has been stripped of its goodness.

• Sugar — too much sugar can depress your immune system. Even table sugar, fructose and honey can cause a 60% drop in the white blood cell's ability to destroy infection.

• Avoid highly processed foods such as microwave dinners. They are often very high in salt and low in essential vitamins. The microwaving process also destroys vitamins. If you want something quick, eat raw. Carrot sticks, cauliflower pieces, nuts and fruit are just a few examples of food that can be eaten raw.

Providing the right environment for your baby to grow

It is important that your Surrogate is given everything that she is going to need to produce a healthy baby for you. This can be helped by buying her the right pre-natal vitamins and mineral supplements that she might benefit from. Even those Surrogates who have led a very healthy lifestyle could do with a little boost. Ask your pharmacist for advice, and invest in the highest quality pre-natal vitamin and mineral supplements that you can afford.

Folic acid is particularly valuable, as it is essential for healthy spine formation. Folic acid may also reduce the risk of other defects, such as cleft lip, cleft palate, and certain heart defects. By taking vitamin B too, a woman can reduce her baby's risk of neural tube defects such as spina bifida and anencephaly by 50 to 70 %.

Iron is another important mineral that should be put on the top of your list. Most Surrogates don't get enough of this mineral in their diet to meet their body's increased need during pregnancy, which can lead to iron-deficiency anaemia. By increasing the Surrogate's iron intake, you can help avoid iron-deficiency anaemia and can cut down risk of pre-term delivery, low birth weight and infant mortality.

5. Getting Pregnant via IVF (Gestational Surrogacy)

What is In Vitro Fertilization (IVF)?

For Gestational Surrogacy (or surrogacy where the Intended Mother's eggs are used), we have to use In Vitro Fertilization or IVF. ("In vitro" meaning "in glass"; i.e. fertilization taking place within a laboratory dish or test tube.) IVF involves stimulating multiple egg follicles, allowing eggs to develop in the ovaries in one woman; then taking the eggs out of that woman; fertilizing them in the laboratory with the Intended Father's (or donated) sperm; and transferring the resulting embryos back to the waiting uterus of another woman, the Gestational Surrogate.

Some lesbian couples use IVF so that an embryo is created with the egg from one partner but is carried by the other partner. This is either due to infertility problems, or so that both partners have been involved in creating the pregnancy.

The first IVF baby in the world, Louise Brown, was born in July 1978 in England, using a technique developed by Drs Edwards and Steptoe in Cambridge. Louise Brown was 28 when she delivered her own baby (conceived without IVF) in 2006. Across the world, thousands of children are now born every year as a result of this technique.

IVF and fertility

In a sense, IVF compresses many months of 'natural' attempts at reproduction into one menstrual cycle, increasing the efficiency of human reproduction. However, IVF is only effective if a woman is able to carry a pregnancy to term, so the Surrogate you use needs to have been screened properly beforehand. The clinic that you use will need to carry out the appropriate testing, normally done by internal examination alongside scans, before IVF treatment proceeds.

It is important to remember that, with surrogacy, neither the Surrogate nor Egg Donor will have fertility problems. Intended Parents may well have been through several IVF attempts themselves, but this will have been due to recognized infertility issues. The chances of success with Gestational Surrogacy are inevitably greater than when treating infertility.

Overall, the chances are high of the first attempt at IVF producing multiple healthy eggs and resulting in healthy embryos, one or more of which will be transferred into the Surrogate's womb three-five days after fertilization. Although many eggs will not fertilize successfully, there is a good chance that there will be embryos remaining after treatment, which can be frozen for future use on day five or six after fertilization. This then circumvents the declining fertility of the Egg Donor herself as she ages, as well as negating the need for the donor to undergo a second cycle of treatment.

It is necessary to understand that, as women age, fewer eggs are produced with IVF. More importantly, we see lower rates of implantation per embryo. The rate of miscarriage also increases with the age of the eggs used. Many Intended Mothers like to have a go with their own eggs, even into their late 30s, but the success rates are not as high as they are when using an egg from a woman in her early to mid 20s. This is why some Intended Parents begin with using eggs from the Intended Mother, but move to using donated eggs instead before pregnancy results.

The IVF Process

The IVF process is very time consuming, and has psychological effects on different women in different ways. For an Intended Mother, who may well have gone through many bouts of IVF herself, seeing another woman go through it on her behalf can be quite overwhelming. For others, the procedure can be exciting and scary at the same time.

In a natural menstrual cycle, only one follicle with one egg inside it is developed, so with IVF the woman who is providing the eggs is stimulated with medications to produce multiple follicles and eggs. When the doctor decides that there are enough follicles, they will organise for the Egg Donor or Intended Mother to come into the clinic. There, using a local anaesthetic, they will retrieve the eggs from the ovaries with the help of a scan machine and a needle.

Once the eggs have been removed, the Embryologist takes over and fertilizes the eggs in a laboratory using sperm from the Intended Father or a donor. The Embryologist will culture the embryos for several days, and then pick the best one (or more than one) for transfer to the Surrogate. It is important for the Embryologist to select the best embryos on the day of transfer, as this increases success rates. The Embryologist and doctor then work together to transfer the embryos to the best location in the middle of the uterus.

This various different stages of the IVF process are described in further detail below.

Choosing an IVF clinic

Your choice of IVF clinic will play a crucial role in the surrogacy process. In the UK, since surrogacy is seen as a relatively new means to treat infertility, not many clinics will have experience in handling the sensitive nature of the surrogacy process. Working with an inexperienced clinic can make for a daunting experience. I have recently seen in my dealings with many of the UK clinics the almost God-like manner in which some of the fertility professionals treat their patients.

I have had Intended Parents come out of meetings with the doctors in tears because they were made to feel as if they had given up on carrying a baby themselves, or that they should come to terms with the fact that they were never meant to become parents if they could not conceive themselves with the help of IVF. I have also seen Surrogates treated in the same way. At a point when the world is going through one of the toughest economic times in living memory, you would think that these facilities would wake up and become more patient-focused, and work with Intended Parents and Surrogates to help to create families at the same time as growing their own businesses.

It will not be long now before we see some of the bigger US-based fertility clinics making moves into Europe. As we develop surrogacy, and our expectations as consumers grow, we will welcome the professionalism of these large American clinics with open arms, and happily watch the demise of some of the clinics that we are currently forced to work with in the UK.

Wherever you live or arrange a surrogacy, when you first make contact with a potential IVF clinic, chat to the receptionist or whoever answers the phone. Ask directly and confidently: "Do you work with Surrogates and Egg Donors?" Most will tell you the truth straightaway, rather than the sales-chat that you will eventually get from the clinic manager or business development head. The manager will often have a deadline to make up the numbers of new clients before their next management meeting, so is more likely to tell you what they think you want to hear than the receptionist is.

You will also need to make sure that you know the success rates of the IVF clinics you are considering using. Most clinics make this easy by posting success rates on their websites or in their monthly newsletters. Also ask them to confirm what percentage of multiple pregnancies they have, and compare these to others. Utilize the free services of to-hatch.co.uk in the UK, where you will find all the statistics that are currently available on success rates. Some clinics are happy with a success rate near the 30-35% mark, but I would not work with a clinic that is not achieving at least 50%. Find out what rates they offer, and if they will give you reduced rates for each attempt you have to go through.

However, it is important to remember that clinics can only post success rates for the types of patients who they are currently working with, and most of these will be couples who are dealing in some way or other with a fertility problem. This can make the success rates look lower than they would actually be if clinics were only working with surrogacy pregnancies where there is no infertility issue. See if it is possible to work out from their stats which were 'healthy' pregnancies and which were not.

If you are still happy at this point, ask for a meeting at the clinic to see what the facility looks like and to meet other people in the waiting area. Talk to waiting patients if possible: ask how their treatment has gone and what they think of the clinic so far. Only decide to work with a clinic once you are entirely happy with everything. Some clinics are busy places, with queues of women and their partners filling up the waiting areas. This can be off-putting to some people, but is a sign that the clinic has a good reputation.

Finding the perfect Egg Donor

Egg Donors are usually young: between 18 years and 35 years. This means that the chances of achieving a pregnancy are much higher and the miscarriage risks statistically less than with Surrogates who have embryos transferred which have been created using older eggs. A 35-year-old Surrogate whose embryo has been created with an egg from a 20-year old will have the same chance of achieving a pregnancy and carrying it to term as a woman who is 15 years younger. It is interesting to note that, since the egg contributes approximately 95% and sperm only 5% to the ultimate 'quality' of the embryo, the Sperm Donor's age is of much less importance.

However, in addition to age, there are a range of other issues to think about when you are looking for an Egg Donor. First you need to think about appearance: do you want your Egg Donor to have the same genetic characteristics as one or more of the Intended Parents? You might also want to look at the Egg Donor's interests, be they musical, artistic, sporting or intellectual (although the jury is still out on how much genetics contribute to any of these interests or achievements).

If one Intended Parent is contributing eggs or sperm to the pregnancy, you may wish to match the Egg Donor as closely as possible with the genetic characteristics of the other Intended Parent. Or if you are a single person, you might want to match the characteristics as closely as possible with yourself (this seems to be the advice given to most single women who are being treated by infertility clinics).

However, there are other issues that are at least as important as appearance and interests. It is very important to look at the medical history of the Egg Donor and her family's overall health, with particular emphasis on infectious diseases, mental health, substance abuse and high rates of cancers, diabetes or heart disease. Look at detailed genetic histories for the whole family where possible, and try to avoid doubling up on possible genetic issues with the person who is contributing the sperm. Obviously, things can and will be missed, but overall most of us have a good understanding of our family genetics and the Egg Donor will be no different.

It is then important for the potential donor to have a thorough ovarian function assessment, including 'FMR1' testing where possible. This is the first blood test for predicting the chances that IVF will lead to a successful pregnancy. A researcher at the Albert Einstein College of Medicine of Yeshiva University helped to develop the test, reported in the online medical journal PLoS One. The test is based on the finding that different subtypes of the FMR1 gene (also known as the Fragile X gene which affects mental development) in potential mothers are associated with significantly different chances of conceiving with IVF.

It is also important for your Egg Donor to have ongoing detailed social evaluations, including of her personality, talents, hobbies and, most importantly, of her motivation for donation. She will need support throughout the donation process, and it's important to offer her counselling so that she can see the importance of what she is doing and feels comfortable with what will happen to her eggs. Donating eggs is a much more complex and emotional process than sperm donation, which until the resulting children were given the right to know the name of their donor (in the UK, not the US), men typically engaged in without giving it a great deal of thought before or afterwards.

You should also think and talk about the amount of involvement you want from your Egg Donor. Do you want to make friends with the donor and have an active interest in each other's lives for the rest of your lives, and then have your future children meet and know the donor as the biological mother? Or do you want an anonymous relationship where you do not even meet the Egg Donor? (In this situation she is known only by a number all the way through the donation, and all you get to see are her medical records and some basic information about her and her immediate family.)

Most people opt for something in between. Certainly the majority of Egg Donors are of the opinion that they would rather donate eggs to a family they have at least met once, or spoken to on the telephone or on Skype if that is not possible. This means that being willing to have at least some contact with your Egg Donor will increase your choice, as well as helping you to find a donor more quickly than otherwise.

Agency benefits

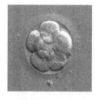

It is getting increasingly difficult to find an Egg Donor now. In the US, big money changes hands when an Egg Donor 'donates' her eggs to a couple. At the opposite end of the spectrum, in the UK only "reasonable expenses" can be paid, which offers women less incentive to volunteer. However, women will always feel more comfortable volunteering via a reputable agency that they can trust to protect their interests and to screen Intended Parents. After registration, the agency will then make contact with them when a selection process has highlighted their profile as a match for a potential couple.

A good agency will have Egg Donors from all walks of life registered on their database. Donors will also be from a wide range of ethnic backgrounds and religions, and will possess a wide array of physical characteristics including eye colour, hair colour, skin tone, height, weight, build, freckles, etc. Most will also offer a choice of talents, such as music, dance, acting or the arts. In addition, most agencies are happy to help you to find a donor with something specific in common with you, such as a shared personal interest or similar life ambitions.

If you are going to find your Egg Donor and Surrogate through an agency, you need to remember that you will have fees for both. This means that if you register with a surrogacy agency, you will pay the registration fees with them (retainer fee), which is anywhere between $8,000-$22,000 depending on which one you go with. Remember also that commercial surrogacy is illegal in the UK, and you cannot pay these fees legally here. The British Surrogacy Centre does not charge a retainer fee or joining fee, and is the only centre of its kind anywhere in the world.

What happens when you have agreed the Egg Donor to work with?

Once you have looked through several profiles and decided on the donor you would like to be matched with, the agency will make contact with her to check that she is available. Each agency will have an Egg Donor Coordinator, whose job it is to recruit new donors and to keep the database of potentials up-to-date with information about previous cycles etc.

Typically, Egg Donors are working with up to three agencies at one time. This means that even though your chosen Donor may not have been matched with Intended Parents through the agency you have chosen to work with, she may still already be matched through another agency.

If the donor is available for the recipient's desired time frame and passes the initial screening as required by the FDA/HFSE with all the blood testing etc, a match is made. During the matching process personal information will often be exchanged with each person involved, such as photos, medical history and anything else deemed appropriate. In some cases, the Egg Donor will request a meeting with the Intended Parents, or visa versa. This could either take place face-to-face, or via the telephone or Skype.

Ovarian stimulation for the Egg Donor

Once the contracts have been signed and all medical screening has taken place, the clinician will put the Egg Donor on to a course of self-administered daily injections of Lupron. These will suppress her natural menstrual cycle, so that it can be synchronized with the recipient's. During the ovarian stimulation phase the donor also uses daily injections of gonadotropins, to stimulate her ovaries. These encourage more than one egg to mature for retrieval. The donor is monitored closely throughout this process, using blood tests and ultrasound scans, to ensure that her ovaries are responding well and are not going into hyper-stimulation (this is a medical complication which in extreme cases can be fatal). Women who have been through an egg retrieval cycle state that self-administering the shots is no more than uncomfortable, and that the procedure is relatively straightforward and easy.

Lining development for the Surrogate

While the Egg Donor is on her medication, the Surrogate will also be taking drugs to stimulate her ovaries. A favourable uterine environment, especially an endometrium (womb lining) depth of at least 7mm, is crucial in the success of an Egg Donor cycle. The Surrogate therefore takes Oestrogen and Progesterone to prepare her endometrial lining for implantation. Developing the endometrium for embryo transfer is usually unproblematic, but in any case the clinician will monitor the developing lining closely during the run-up to transfer for its suitability to accept the developing embryos.

Egg retrieval

Timing is crucial in an IVF cycle. The clinicians will monitor the Egg Donor over a two-week period, and will decide on the day when egg retrieval is going to take place. Blood samples may be taken to measure response to ovarian stimulation medications. Normally, Oestrogen levels increase as the follicles develop, while Progesterone levels are low until after ovulation.

Generally, eight to 14 days after starting the injections, the medical professionals will need to take a look at what's going on in the ovaries. A scan will confirm that the eggs have sufficiently developed, after which the donor will be instructed to trigger ovulation with an injection of HCG hormone. Approximately 36 hours before retrieval, the donor must administer this last injection of HCG to ensure that her eggs are ready to be harvested. Two days later, the eggs will be removed during a short procedure called egg retrieval. The donor is put to sleep using simple intravenous sedation, while an aspiration needle, guided by ultrasound, is used transvaginally to aspirate (remove) the eggs. This is achieved by connecting the needle to a suction device.

Removal of multiple eggs can usually be completed in less than 30 minutes. However, there are some circumstances where one or both ovaries may not be accessible by transvaginal ultrasound. Then laparoscopy will be used to retrieve the eggs instead, using a small telescope placed in the umbilicus.

Fertilization and Embryo Transfer

Once the eggs are retrieved from the donor by the doctor, the embryologist will begin the process of fertilizing them. At this point the frozen sample of semen will be ready and waiting. (Fresh semen is not normally used because of the risk of infection; however, if all parties are happy with it, it is up to the clinician.) Depending on which procedure is called for with the fertilization, the embryologist will add the prepared sperm to each egg, and they will then be allowed to incubate overnight under controlled laboratory conditions. The following day each egg is evaluated for evidence of fertilization.

In some cases no eggs will have been fertilized, or only a few of them will have been — this is particularly the case when the eggs have come from an older woman. However, the hope is that at least half have fertilized, which will allow two or more attempts at implantation and therefore a better chance of achieving at least one pregnancy.

The resulting embryos are then incubated and graded. Two days after egg retrieval, a fertilized egg will have divided to become a 2- to 4-cell embryo. By the third day, a normally developing embryo will contain approximately 6-10 cells. By the fifth day, a fluid cavity forms in the embryo, and the placenta and foetal tissues begin to separate. An embryo at this stage is called a blastocyst.

Within the blastocyst there are two types of cells. In the interior of the blastocyst is the inner cell mass. A portion of the cells in this mass will soon begin to divide at a very rapid pace indeed to become the developing foetus. The inner cell mass is surrounded by a fluid-filled cavity called the blastocoel. Surrounding this is a single layer of cells called the trophoblast, which will combine with the endometrial cells of the uterus to become the placenta. The embryologist will be monitoring the developing embryos on a daily basis and grading each one individually.

When they are judged to be at their peak, the embryologist will inform the clinician and they will set the time to transfer one or more into the Surrogate's uterus. The hope will be that successful development continues in the uterus, and that the embryo hatches from the surrounding zona pellucida which will then implant into the lining of the uterus. Some doctors think that transferring blastocysts, which are five days old, is more effective, because they tend to be more stable than three-day-old embryos. Around half of embryos do not reach day five of development anyway, so by transferring five-day-old embryos there is a greater chance that the embryo will remain viable after transfer and a successful pregnancy will result.

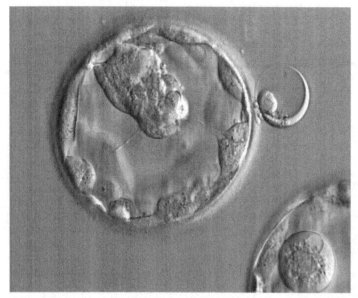

A BLASTOCYST

Embryo transfer

This is a relatively painless procedure and no anaesthesia is necessary, although some women choose to have a mild sedative in order to help them relax a little. Once the Gestational Surrogate is in position, the embryologist will draw one or two embryos into a transfer catheter, a long, thin sterile tube with a syringe on one end. This is then gently guided through the woman's cervix and placed into the uterine cavity. The number of embryos transferred is largely based on the age of

Egg Donor, but usually two embryos are transferred at a time. Any pregnancy which involves more than two babies is considered to be high-risk, which no one wants to deal with.

Freezing remaining embryos

Normally, there are several embryos remaining that can then be frozen. These can be used for future attempts if the first, fresh cycle, did not work, or if you want siblings at a later date. Once frozen, embryos may be stored for several years.

Embryo thawing

Embryo thawing involves warming the embryos to room temperature and takes approximately two hours. The embryos are thawed either the day before or on the day of the scheduled embryo transfer.

Some embryos survive the freezing and thawing process and some do not; there is currently at least no way to predict this in advance. Sometimes individual cells within the embryo are damaged by the freezing process. Embryos with some freeze damage can still go on to produce a healthy pregnancy; however, the more the embryo is damaged, the less likely it is to develop. If all of the cells are damaged, the embryo cannot be transferred.

6. Working with Professionals

The number of professionals involved in a surrogate pregnancy, and when they are involved, will depend on the type of surrogacy that you opt for. With Traditional Surrogacy, which often takes place between friends or relatives, few professionals are involved from the start. You meet someone, agree the terms between yourselves, then start Home Inseminations with the hope of becoming pregnant and then taking delivery of the baby. If insemination is taking place at a clinic, there should be clinic-specific rules on what their protocols call for in terms of counselling and blood testing etc. However, the unfortunate truth is that few people opting for co-parenting situations or Traditional Surrogacy bother to do any checks or opt for counselling beforehand.

There are some professionals that you really should be working with, though. These include lawyers to help with the parental agreements, as well as submissions to the Home Office if these are also needed to establish you as the parents. As discussed in Chapter 4., blood tests should always be carried out before Home Inseminations to screen for HIV and the like, and these will involve doctors and other medical professionals.

Counselling should be offered to your Surrogate before insemination begins, during pregnancy and for at least three months after the birth, so that she is cared for properly and her mental and physical needs are met. It is also helpful for you to have established contact with a counsellor yourselves, since emotional issues might well arise that you have not anticipated. And you will inevitably come into contact with social services along the way, and it is much better to plan and thus control this process yourself (see below).

It is completely different for those of you who are going to be using a Gestational Surrogate. From your decision to go forward, you will be surrounded by professionals for the entire journey.

Working with an agency

If you decide to work with an agency, then they will be organising most of the meetings and appointments that you and your Surrogate and Egg Donor will need. Otherwise, you will need to organize these for yourself.

If you work with an agency, a caseworker who will be assigned to you. They will be there with you throughout the process, and will be able to give you sound advice on the steps that you need to take to organise your surrogacy in accordance with the laws of the country you are living in. (If the caseworker is not conversant with country specific issues relating to your surrogacy, then you should change agencies.)

The caseworker will also be responsible for your timetable, and for introducing you to prospective Egg Donors and Surrogates. They will also ensure that your

Surrogate and Egg Donor have had all of the checks that they need to go through before they start working with you, including the country concerned's equivalent to a Criminal Record Bureau (CRB) check. The caseworker will also organize the Surrogate's and Egg Donor's blood tests, which will involve them in trips to the clinic and calls to you from nursing staff and explanations about results from doctors. Psychologists, too, will be involved throughout the process, talking to your Egg Donor and Surrogate and then with you.

If your Surrogate's pregnancy will be taking place in the UK, your caseworker will also be preparing a case report that will be sent to the IVF clinic's Ethics Committee, as they will need to grant approval for your surrogacy. Although this is a well-intentioned process, in reality it is a pointless exercise. There is currently not enough experience in the UK about the issues surrounding surrogacy for a suitably knowledgeable panel of people to be appointed and for them to be able to make an informed decision.

In my experience, clinics want to show that they are following good practice guidelines, but in the process they tend to waste time waiting for Ethics Committees to be formed and meet — meetings which inevitably get rescheduled continuously throughout the year with no prior warning. At best, this tends to make Intended Parents, Surrogates and Egg Donors uneasy. For those Intended Parents who have already have been waiting for many years to get pregnant, delays caused by Ethics Committees encourage them to go overseas, where in some countries, as previously discussed, ethical concerns about the welfare of the Surrogate and resulting children may be non-existent.

In any case, the professionals that you will see throughout a Gestational Surrogacy are:

- Your agency's caseworker
(if you are working with an agency)
- Social worker (country specific)
- Phlebotomist (nurse for blood tests)
- IVF doctor
- Psychologist/counsellor
- IVF nurse
- Hospital delivery nurse
- Hospital delivery doctor
- Hospital social worker
- Hospital registry workers
- Lawyers (to establish parental responsibility)
- Local Passport Office
(if baby is born outside of your country)

Along the way, and depending on what complications you might experience, there may be additional professionals who you come into contact with as well.

Social Workers

The British Surrogacy Centre is unique in that we attach a social worker to each of our cases. Their role is to make sure that you have all the information you need to make an informed decision. Ultimately, the social worker is responsible for the welfare of any children born through surrogacy, and it is their job to ensure that children born through surrogacy have good homes rather than ending up in local social services care.

The social worker will arrange all of the checks on you that are needed to go forward with the British

Surrogacy Centre: these include an enhanced CRB check. This will tell the social worker if you have any convictions that would normally rule you out of a fostering or adoptive situation. Old petty convictions are something that your social worker will talk to you about, but in my experience would not be enough to rule you out. The social worker will, though, need to be convinced that you are the right people to enter into a surrogacy arrangement, and that the resulting child/ren will be looked after properly in the home where they will ultimately spend their life.

The social worker will also seek professionals to work on your case who will give you good value for money, but who have worked in the area of surrogacy for some time. (The worst thing you can do is to work with an agency without any experience of surrogacy, because you will end up being their test case and you will pay heavily for the privilege.) They will also work with you to complete the paperwork needed to establish your parental rights, and to amend the birth certificate to show both the Intended Parents' names.

During the course of Traditional or self-organised Gestational Surrogacies, social workers were never involved professionally before the opening of the British Surrogacy Centre. In reality, anyone, regardless of their past criminal convictions, has been able to hire a Surrogate around the world and have a baby. The needs of the child have not been taken into account, and ultimately, if this is allowed to continue, we will be seeing children born through surrogacy placed into local social services' care.

Even though you might not use a social worker in the UK, hospitals around the world do. With this in mind, social workers in hospital environments are on the look out for anything out of the ordinary. Certainly in the US, where babies' birth certificates are prepared by hospitals before being sent off to vital record departments, social workers are more aware of surrogacies as they happen than in the UK, where most of the arrangements are done without the knowledge of the hospital or the social work team there.

For years, people's preference has always been not not to involve social workers within the process of surrogacy, for fear that the child may end up in social services care. This is just not correct. True, most social workers are not experienced enough in the UK to deal with the issues surrounding surrogacy, and this needs to be addressed in their training. However, social workers are not trying to take children away, but rather to make sure that they are adequately looked after by the right people. The welfare of any child born through a surrogacy situation is paramount to all the professionals involved, and this will normally be best protected through living with the Intended Parents.

Medical screening and counselling

Medical screening is a must-do if you are organizing things yourself. As I discussed earlier, it is important that you get all the STD testing needed carried out before you try to have a baby. If the Surrogate is not clear of STDs, then she may pass something on to your baby. If the Intended Father is infected with HIV, for example, he may pass this on to the Surrogate. The British Surrogacy Centre can organize all your testing needs regardless of whether they are helping you with your surrogacy. The professionals there will be able to do all the testing needed, and also offer the Surrogate the counseling that she will need, even though she will try to convince you that you don't need to waste your money on it. You really do.

It's important to try to establish if the woman who may become your Surrogate is mentally and physically in the best condition that she can be to get pregnant, and then to maintain a healthy pregnancy throughout the term of that pregnancy. You also need to be sure that she is ready in her own mind to give up the baby when it is born.

It's also important to remember that the baby born through Traditional Surrogacy is the biological baby of the woman giving birth. It takes a very special woman to be able to give up her own baby, and you need to make sure that she is ready to do this in the best way possible. Of course, nothing is ever certain and people do change their minds, but you must do everything you can to make sure that she is already reconciled to her loss in nine months time.

Be guided by the experts. Even if you wish to find your own Surrogate and Egg Donor, if you have a friend or family member who has said that they will do it for you, do the right thing and get them the help that they will certainly need going forward.

The Birth

When it comes to the birth part of the surrogacy, it's important to get to know the people you will see when the birth approaches. In the US, you will have seen the delivering doctor throughout the pregnancy. In the UK, it could be whoever is on duty in the hospital at the time. You should try to be as open with the staff there as possible to avoid any issues later.

What you tell the people in the hospital is up to you. I have always thought that honesty is the best policy. You have nothing to hide: what you are doing is not illegal in some countries; and I hope is certainly not illegal in the country you are planning to live in. With this in mind, be open about the arrangement that you have with your Surrogate. Let the team who are looking after her, and who will be looking after your baby, know that you are the parents, and that after the birth the child(ren) will be in your care. If you are in the US, the birthing hospital will already know and so will the social work department, as they will have had a copy of the Parental Order to make sure that your names go on the birth certificate.

In my experience, most people want to be as private about their surrogacy as possible. The reality is, though, that there are people that you have to work with to make it happen. The old saying of "If I could clone myself..." goes out the window, because if you could clone yourself, you would be in the same position, without a child! Think about the list of professionals mentioned in the other chapters of this book and how you will bring them together. They are all there to provide services for you, you just need to know how to use them.

Comment to professionals: It's hard enough for any couple to have to find someone else to come into their relationship and help them to achieve something that most of their family members can do quite naturally. Many are at the point of desperation, knowing that they are never going to be parents without the help of a Surrogate or an Egg Donor, and they are at breaking point. Remember the grief that many have been through on their journey: some have buried children; and others have never achieved a pregnancy despite years of trying. Some have "unexplained" infertility, nothing is worse than not knowing why. At least when a condition is diagnosed, you can say "well, that's why..."

Remember your training: inclusive services for all, regardless of all the obvious things like age, colour and sexual orientation. Be progressive within your own profession, and challenge the comments of team mates who do not like the sound of surrogacy, or who have no compassion for those people who find themselves using the services that they have a right to use.

As a professional in your own area, you know what is right and wrong. A teacher is there to teach the child in their care, not to judge the actions of the parent. The medical professional should be able to see past their own prejudices and offer the treatment necessary to get the Surrogate pregnant for the Intended Parents, without the attitude and the pomposity that so many of them display.

What is the role of the Ethics Committee at the fertility clinic in terms of a surrogacy arrangement?

The purpose of the Medical Ethics Committee at a fertility clinic is to support families and hospital staff in the resolution of ethical issues that may occur in the course of hospitalization and treatment. Surrogacy was not generally thought about when these committees were set up, but is now automatically referred to them within the UK. The Committee meets in a private room, and discusses your case on a case-by-case basis. They will have been sent all your case files, including the report that the Psychologist has put together after her meetings with you over the past two months or so.

The main role of the Medical Ethics Committee is to review specific, individual patient-care situations and dilemmas. After the review, the Committee provides an opinion about the situation from an ethical point of view. The consultation process aims to assist all those involved in having an open discussion about the Intended Parent's reason for their infertility. The outcome of the consult is a recommendation about which course of action would be in the Intended Parents', Surrogate's and, if needed, the Egg Donor's best interests.

The members of the Medical Ethics Committee come from a wide variety of medical and non-medical fields within the hospital and community. Professionals who work at the hospital, such as doctors, nurses, social workers, ethicists, and chaplains, serve with a diverse group of community clergy, attorneys, and interested citizens. The physicians and nurses on the committee represent a variety of clinical specialties, such as Internal Medicine, Neurology, Neurosurgery, Psychiatry, fertility, Cardiology, and Intensive Care. However, it is interesting to note that few of these committees in the UK have members who have gone through IVF, let alone surrogacy.

I have helped many couples and singles over the years to meet Surrogates and Egg Donors who have had their medical procedures performed in the UK. The benefit of this is that the treatment in the UK is second to none. After all, IVF was created and established here in the UK before it was carried out anywhere else in the world. However, the care of patients in any hospital is increasingly complex, and with a surrogacy there is inevitably additional stress. The need to go to a Medical Ethics Committee before any of the work actually starts adds more pressure to all concerned, without their decisions being based on enough evidence and experience to be of particular value.

I have often found it hard to understand what on earth qualifies some of these people to sit in judgment on anyone who wants to use surrogacy as a way of having a baby. Often, their involvement appears to be a paper exercise to make it appear that due diligence is being carried out. Doctors and clinics will, in any case, use their professional judgment before taking on a patient for treatment. They will also refer a case to an Ethics Committee if they feel that it merits it. I feel that otherwise these committees should NOT be involved in the decision process, and that the confidential aspects of each case should not be discussed by people who are not directly involved with the process simply for the sake of it.

What also concerns me is the irregularity of the meetings, and in some cases the fact that one or two lead members of the committee can put the meetings back by several months because of personal issues that come up for them. This adds to the stress being experienced by the Surrogate and Intended Parents, as well as affecting the timing and planning of treatments. If a member of the committee cannot be present for whatever reason, the meeting should go ahead with the rest of them.

I would argue that, if a responsible adult wants to use surrogacy as an option for having a baby and all parties involved are consenting, and the medical professionals are happy that the Surrogate is medically and mentally fit to be pregnant and carry a healthy pregnancy, then the decision to go forward should be left with the treating fertility expert. A quick review by ten strangers who have had no personal dealings with the people involved should not be allowed to affect that decision. It would never happen for the majority of other IVF cases, and it certainly does not happen for those people who are arranging a Traditional Surrogacy using Home Inseminations.

7. Using a Surrogate Overseas

"We had considered adoption and even fostering as an option, and did meet with a social
worker from an agency, but felt that the
process was not for us at all. We decided, after
much research, that we would look for an
agency that would take us through the process
of surrogacy from start to finish. We met with
many different agency reps throughout the US
and India, but felt unsure about them being
over 5000 miles away. When we realised that
we could go through the process with a centre
in the UK, and that they would manage everything locally in the US for us, we decided to use
the British Surrogacy Centre. We are currently
expecting Boy/Girl twins, and looking forward
to the birth in December."

Sean and Gavin, Birmingham, UK

Without surrogacy, many of us would never have had
the chance to have had children. We remain, to this day,
forever humbled by the chances that surrogacy has
given to us. There is no doubt that many countries have

strict policies on surrogacy. Some ban it outright, while others tolerate it to a certain degree but regulate it to some degree or other. With this in mind, you should try to work out how much time away from home you are going to have to commit to, first to get your Surrogate pregnant, and then to wait once the babies are born to bring them home. In the USA we say you only need to take three trips: one to freeze sperm and meet the clinic staff; the second at week 20 of the pregnancy to see what you are having; and the third to collect your baby.

Of course, the amount of time you need to stay abroad for each visit is different. For the first visit, we say fly out on a Thursday afternoon, meet the clinic staff on Friday morning and leave your sample, and fly back Saturday for arrival back in the UK on Sunday and return to work on Monday! Your second visit really is optional. You may do it because it's great to see your baby on the screen, and you get to meet the Surrogate properly. If not, the final visit will be to collect the baby/ies, and the waiting period will be for the birth certificate(s) and passport(s) to arrive. The shortest time for this is about three weeks. You must also check with the airline you plan to use to see how old a baby has to be to fly with them.

The options

There are a number of countries around the world that have, during the past five years, developed into meccas for desperate childless couples and singles to go in search of a Surrogate Mother and Egg Donor. At the time of writing, the most popular of these are Thailand,

India, Ukraine, the UK and the US. This is not an exhaustive list, but these are the most popular places for foreigners to go to for surrogacy, so for the sake of this book I have only concentrated on them.

Thailand

Thailand's reputation as a place where Surrogate Mothers can be found easily and cheaply is growing. Thai Surrogate Mothers are well regarded for their healthy lifestyle, and for the low fees that they charge. As a rule, Surrogates in Thailand are paid a fee of around £6000 ($9,600) for carrying a surrogate baby. This is almost five years' salary for a poor rural Thai family: one surrogacy can boost the family's income 100-fold.

Thailand also has a first-class hospital system, and there is no doubt that the IVF clinics there are world-class too. Thai private hospitals are extremely welcoming to visitors from overseas, as they bring with them the funds to maintain facilities which otherwise could not exist. It is unsurprising that hundreds of childless couples flock there each year to begin the surrogacy process when they are so welcomed to do so. In particular, Thailand has become a very popular destination for Australian same-sex couples, and for many German couples too.

The ugly side of surrogacy in Thailand

However, it is not all good news. As Westerners have gone to Thailand in ever-larger numbers, there have been many reports over the past few years of families selling their unmarried daughters to teams of recruiters. These drive around the poorer areas of Thailand convincing families to part with their daughters, and in some cases husbands to part with their wives, for a year to act as a Surrogate for a Western couple. As a result, there have been scandals regarding rings of pimps and gangs who have set up houses in Bangkok and other areas with women who have been 'bought' or 'rented' in this way. Gangs and pimps have also been known to bring women in across the Vietnamese borders to give birth for Western couples.

In February 2011, police in Thailand announced that they had rescued 14 Vietnamese women aged between 19-26 from a criminal "baby breeding" ring. The women had been promised money in return for being Surrogate Mothers, but once they arrived in Thailand they had their passports confiscated and were told that they would be given half the agreed fee once they had delivered a baby to the Intended Parent couples. The Thai police arrested four Taiwanese, one Chinese and three Burmese nationals in connection with the operation.

At the time of writing, Thai authorities are still trying to decide what to do with the offspring of the Vietnamese women. A total of 14 women, half of them pregnant, were freed but put into a holding house until the courts could decide what to do with them. The baby sales operation had used the women as Surrogates for wealthy childless couples overseas who had literally placed orders for newborns online. Most of the women had never met the couples who they were having the babies for, nor had they had any telephone conversations with them. The babies have been born into a legal grey area, with Thailand still mulling over the ramifications of the case.

Six of the babies that have been born so far are now in a care home in Bangkok. Three have had their Intended Parents identified, but police are finding it hard to trace the parents of the other three children. No paperwork had been kept, and the Intended Parents had had no contact with the Surrogate so she could not let them know that she had given birth. What made it particularly difficult is that in some European countries, such as France, surrogacy is illegal, so the Intended Parents may not have wanted to come forward because of the legal ramifications. The babies will remain in the care home until new, suitable parents can be found for them.

Surrogacy law in Thailand

It was only recently that legislation was put in place to help protect the rights of the woman being used within surrogacy in Thailand. In recognition of the legal minefield that can arise in these difficult situations, the Thai Cabinet has now approved draft legislation for children born through the use of Assisted Reproductive Technologies (ART) including surrogacy. The draft surrogacy law covers two types of surrogacy:

1. Where a married couple uses their own egg and

sperm, but the child is carried by someone else.

2. Where a Surrogate Mother provides an egg and carries the child, but the fertilising sperm comes from either a donor or the commissioning parent.

As in many countries, including the UK, under Thai law the birth mother is recognised as the mother of that child. Since 90% of Thai Surrogates are usually married, a child born as a result of surrogacy will be registered as the child of the Surrogate Mother and her husband. Hence, under current Thai law, the Intended Parents have no automatic legal rights. It is therefore crucial that both the birth mother and her husband actively renounce their rights to the child. Should you need to go to a court in Thailand, Thai surrogacy law says that the Juvenile and Family Court will be given authority for judging paternity.

Draft surrogacy law proposals actually do set out some protection for the Thai Surrogate Mother. The draft law states that the Surrogate Mother must be married and that her husband must also give consent to the surrogacy process, especially to the use of sperm from another man. This is clearly important in reducing the likelihood that the Surrogate and her family will claim any rights over the child when it is born.

It is advised to set out a contract with the Surrogate in Thailand, although it is still unclear whether or not the courts would uphold a contract if a dispute were to arise. However, having a contract will show that there was at the least the intent to pass the child at birth to the Intended Parents. As discussed earlier, wherever you perform your surrogacy it is best to set up a contract with your Surrogate, just so that you can show that the intent was always there even in a country where a surrogacy contract would not be enforceable.

When thinking about using a potential Thai

Surrogate, you should employ prudence. Significant legal issues can still arise — not least in respect of taking the child out of Thailand if the commissioning parents are from overseas. This is still a grey area, and one that is changing all the time. Currently there isn't a clear process for the Intended Parents to obtain a Pre-Birth Order in Thailand to establish their parental rights.

Intended Parents also need to remember that they are going to have to go through an adoption process, which will inevitably involve interaction with the Thai authorities. With this in mind it is important that you get as much legal advice as possible to avoid a situation where you have broken the law and cannot take your child out of the country.

India

India's 'reproductive tourism' industry is growing rapidly and is now a $450 million-a-year industry. Presently there is a bill under consideration in the Indian parliament that purports to regulate Assisted Reproductive Techniques (ART). Provisions include full information disclosure to Surrogates, such as medical side-effects and risks; minimum-age stipulations; and limits on the number of eggs to be implanted per cycle. The current draft is a clear improvement over the heavily gendered and patriarchal system originally proposed and strongly criticized by women's health advocates in India. This presumed participants to be in heterosexual marriages, and required their husband's permission to be a Surrogate or have IVF treatment.

At present, National Guidelines have been drafted

by an Expert Committee to regulate such activities, anticipating that surrogacy agreements might be favoured as a viable option to fulfill the wishes of infertile couples. The National Guidelines for the Accreditation, Supervision and Regulation of Assisted Reproductive Techniques (ART) clinics in India have not defined either a commercial or an altruistic surrogacy arrangement. Nowhere has the term 'altruistic' been used: these Guidelines have only stated that the ART clinics shall not play a role in commercial surrogacy arrangements.

The National Guidelines are definitely not averse to payments being paid to Surrogates. In fact they are fairly liberal, since they provide for a clause where liability is imposed on the infertile couple to bear the genuine medical expenses. Surprisingly, they even entitle the Surrogate to receive compensation for the service she provides, and provide scope for a private financial agreement to be drawn up between the parties in such circumstances. The Guidelines require documentary evidence of such monetary agreements, as in the UK, i.e. an agreement for genuine expenses or compensation to the Surrogate.

Moreover, the National Guidelines have taken a startlingly different view, compared to other nations, with regard to the issue of participation of close friends and relatives in altruistic arrangements. They prohibit close members of the infertile couple's family from acting as Surrogates. They do not even permit donation of sperm or eggs by such persons, since the ART clinics are responsible for obtaining these from authorized places.

The Guidelines further lay down that an HIV positive woman shall not be refused treatment by ART clinics. Instead, she should be redirected to appropriate counselling service centres where she shall be informed about the potential hazards it may cause to the unborn child, but nevertheless, she shall have the right to treatment.

Same-sex couples in Indian surrogacy arrangements

It is worth noting that at this time only heterosexual couples will be recognized for surrogacy in India. This is because homosexuality and same-sex partnership are illegal in India. The only loophole is that the Draft Bill allows for 'singles' to commission a surrogate pregnancy. Assuming that this legislation is passed in the form drafted by the ICMR, then gay couples presenting themselves as singles will still have the option to use India for their surrogacy. However, those presenting themselves as couples will run into trouble with the Indian bureaucracy.

There are many clinics which may be sympathetic and accommodating, but they are only one part of the equation. Obtaining exit visas for the baby will be outside the scope of the clinics, and the process will follow whatever legislation is on the books. If you present yourself as a single man or woman but are really in a same-sex partnership, you will need to tread very carefully with all the paperwork and take care not to be found out. Please take full legal advice from a legal professional if at all possible.

There have been dozens of couples (if not more) from various countries over the past five years who are currently stranded in India. This is because they did not carry out due diligence regarding citizenship and Indian laws before engaging their respective clinics. It is clear that the clinics are quite good at getting people their babies, but once 'delivered' they disappear into the background very quickly. They do not offer any assistance to their clients in getting the babies out of India if there is some kind of complication.

As with Thailand, there have been problems in India too with pimps buying or leasing women from communities all over India to get them pregnant. Families and women often participate in surrogacy in the hope of taking their families out of poverty. Indian Surrogates get paid around £3500-£5000 ($5617- $8,025), and for some women this is more money than they will ever see in their lifetime. Not all of the women that are involved in the surrogacy process are willing participants, and some have been forced to take part by cruel husbands or other family members.

If you are thinking about India as a place to have your baby, then please use a reputable agency to find your Egg Donor and Surrogate.

USA

The USA has been seen as the land of opportunities for many people for the past couple of hundred years. It certainly was the only option available for the author of this book when he was looking to build his family with his partner. When all other doors were closing, 5500 miles away one door was opening: CALIFORNIA. Surrogacy law is complex, though, and varies from State to State. Some States are extremely surrogacy friendly; others are absolutely no-go areas.

In Michigan and the District of Columbia (D.C), surrogacy contracts are illegal, and parties to the contract can face a $10,000 fine or be jailed for a year. This includes the Intended Parents and the Surrogate, and the Surrogate's husband if she is married. Eleven States prohibit surrogacy agreements in all or some instances.

Some other States allow surrogacy, but regulate it differently. The District of Columbia and Florida prohibit surrogacy for all unmarried couples; Indiana and Louisiana prohibit Traditional Surrogacy; Michigan and Nebraska prohibit compensated surrogacy agreements; Nevada, New York, North Dakota, Utah, Virginia and Texas prohibit surrogacy for all unmarried couples. Where same-sex couples cannot legally marry (the majority of US States), these laws would make it impossible for them to carry out a surrogacy arrangement.

Six States allow individuals and couples to enter into surrogacy contracts: Arkansas, California, Illinois (Gestational Surrogacy only), Massachusetts, New Jersey (altruistic i.e. uncompensated surrogacy agreements only) and Washington (altruistic surrogacy agreements only).

I discuss as many different States as I can below in more detail, with emphasis on those States that the British Surrogacy Centre would recommend. However, when you have met a Surrogate who you wish to work with, it is important to research for yourself what her home State — the State that she is currently living in — thinks about surrogacy. The law is forever changing, so keep an eye on what's new and what's about to happen in each State. You don't want to be half-way through a pregnancy when you have to move your Surrogate out of State for the remainder of it because her State has changed policy on what it will and won't allow.

California Surrogacy Law

California is accepting of surrogacy agreements and upholds agreements that include Lesbian, Gay, Bisexual and Transgender (LGBT) individuals. While the State has no Statute directly addressing surrogacy, California's courts have used the State's Uniform Parentage Act to interpret several cases concerning surrogacy agreements. In fact, one of the most influential cases in the country regarding surrogacy rights (Johnson v. Calvert) was decided in California.

In 1993, the California Supreme Court decided Johnson v. Calvert, in which they held that the Intended Parents in a Gestational Surrogacy agreement (where the Surrogate is not the biological contributor of the egg) should be recognized as the natural and legal parents. The Court decided that the person who intended to procreate — in this case, the mother who provided her egg to the Surrogate — should be considered the natural mother. This also follows through to a couple who uses the services of an Egg Donor.

In the 1994 case of the marriage of Moschetta, a California Court of Appeals addressed the question of how to determine parentage when a child is conceived via Traditional Surrogacy (in which the Surrogate Mother is the biological contributor of the egg) and is born after the Intended Parents had separated. The Court held that the Intended Father and the Surrogate Mother were the legal parents of the child, leaving the Intended Mother without parental rights.

The 1998 case of the marriage of Buzzanca is an example of how complex the facts in surrogacy cases can get. In Buzzanca, a Gestational Surrogate was impregnated using an anonymous egg and anonymous sperm. In other words, one could identify six individuals as having the potential to be a legal parent of the child: the Egg Donor, the Sperm Donor, the Intended Mother, the Intended Father, the gestational mother and the husband of the gestational mother. Ultimately, the Court found that when a married couple intends to procreate using a non-genetically related embryo implanted into a Surrogate, the Intended Parents are the lawful parents of the child.

In 1998, the case of Drewitt-Barlow v Bellamy, a same-sex couple from Essex UK who petitioned the Supreme Court of California for both their names to be assigned to their unborn twin babies' birth certificates when they were born as Parent 1 and Parent 2, was won. This was a landmark case for European couples that paved the way for same-sex couples throughout Europe to be named on their babies' birth certificates; it also had obvious benefits for heterosexual couples.

Finally, in 2005 the California Supreme Court decided three companion cases that concerned lesbian couples who had reproduced via surrogacy: Elisa B. v. Superior Court; Kristine H. v. Lisa R.; and K.M. v. E.G. The Court held that, under the Uniform Parentage Act, two women can be the legal parents of a child produced through surrogacy. This ruling presumably applies to all members of the LGBT community.

One of the most important advantages of performing surrogacy in California is that it is possible to get a Pre-Birth Order that will establish you as the legal parents of any children born to your Surrogate within a specified time period. The time frame to obtain a judgment can take several months, mostly due to the court's availability to review the documents and/or set the matter for hearing. To obtain the Pre-Birth Order, the paperwork would usually be filed with the court between the fourth and seventh month of your

Surrogate's pregnancy. This is now seen as a very standard application. Some states will require that you attend the hearing, others will not.

However, if your Surrogate becomes high risk for early delivery at any point of the pregnancy, for example if your Surrogate is pregnant with multiples, you may choose to file earlier. This is in order to ensure the judgment is in place prior to the birth of your child(ren), to prevent the Surrogate's name from being listed on your child's birth certificate.

Once the Order is obtained, the hospital where your Surrogate will be delivering should be forwarded a copy. Normally this will go to the social work department. This will highlight to the hospital team that this is a surrogacy arrangement, and that specialised handling should be put in place to accommodate the needs of the Intended Parents and the Surrogate and her family. Most hospitals are now very familiar with these arrangements, and have a specific protocol in place to ensure that åthe transition goes smoothly for everyone. Please make sure you have a copy of the judgement with you at all times, as this will help speed things along if the hospital has mislaid or lost the original one they had.

In the US, it is the hospital's duty to register the birth of any children born at that hospital. This means that a full-time registrar will be attached to the hospital, who will come along to your private room within 24 hours of the birth of your babies and fill out the birth registration forms. This form will be signed by you both, and by the delivering doctor. Once this has been done, the registrar will forward the paperwork to the California State Department of Vital records, where the birth certificate will be produced. This will then be ready for collection within the next two weeks.

Birth Certificates in the US — a view from Thomas M. Pinkerton

Thomas M. Pinkerton is recognised as one of the leading and most influential lawyers on the subject of surrogacy anywhere in the US. He has successfully gained Pre-Birth Orders for many couples dating back to the late 1990s, when they were first introduced. In a recent article addressing the issues surrounding birth certificates he said:

"In all cases where a Surrogate gives birth to a child for another couple or person, the California Office of Vital Records will only allow the Intended Parents' name(s) to go on the birth certificate if the certificate is accompanied by a Superior Court judgment naming the Intended Parent(s) as the legal parent(s) of the child. Without such a judgment, the Surrogate's name (and if she is married, her husband's name) must go on the birth certificate. Because the birth certificate must be registered with the Office of Vital Records within ten days of the birth, the judgment should be presented to the birth records department of the hospital at the time of birth. As a practical matter, the judgment should be obtained no later than twenty weeks into the pregnancy. The practical reason for this advice is that after twenty weeks Vital Records will require either a certificate of birth or foetal death, both of which require the parent's name(s).

"Where there is both an Intended Mother and an Intended Father, filling out the birth certificate is straightforward. The hospital where the child is born simply follows the court judgment and fills out the birth certificate with the Intended Mother and Intended Father's names in the appropriate boxes. If a single man is the sole parent, however, the box designated "Mother" cannot be left blank. This means that the single male parent has two choices. He can opt to have the Surrogate's name go in the box for "Mother" and his name in the box for "Father", or he can elect to have his name go in the box for "Mother" and leave the box for "Father" left blank. In both cases, the judgment calls for the birth certificate to be reissued with the single man's name in the box for "Father", and the box for "Mother" left with a dash (-). The best choice is to have his name go in the box for "Mother", so that the birth certificate is as accurate as possible from the time of birth.

"For the gay or lesbian couple, the best course of action is to have the court issue its judgment requiring that both Intended Parents' names go on the birth certificate, one in the box for "Father" and one in the box for "Mother".

New York Surrogacy Law

Since 1992, Surrogate parenting contracts in New York have been seen as void, unenforceable and contrary to public policy. The main reason for this is because surrogacy contracts have been interpreted to involve, in the words of one New York court, the "trafficking of children". The Statute defines Surrogate parenting contracts as agreements in which a Surrogate agrees to be either impregnated with the fertilized ovum of another woman or artificially inseminated; and further agrees to consent to the adoption of the child born as a result of the impregnation or insemination. Parties to surrogate parenting contracts involving compensation are subject to civil penalties of up to $500. The stiffest penalties — fines of up to $10,000 and forfeiture of fees received in connection with such contracts — are levelled against those who arrange compensated surrogacy contracts for profit. Repeat violators of the Statute may be charged with a felony. Parties to uncompensated surrogacy contracts are not subject to civil or criminal penalties.

People who assist in arranging the contract (agencies or facilitators) are liable for up to a civil penalty of $10,000 and forfeiture of the fee received in brokering the contract. A second violation constitutes a felony. A birth mother's participation in the contract, however, may not be held against her in a custody dispute with the genetic parents or grandparents.

Florida Surrogacy Law

Florida law explicitly allows both Gestational Surrogacy agreements and Traditional Surrogacy, but neither are available to same-sex couples. This is because the Florida Gestational Surrogacy Statutes impose strict requirements on the contracts, among them limiting involvement to "couples that are legally married [which then prevents same-sex couples from being allowed to use surrogacy as they are not legally married] and are both 18 years of age or older." The law governing Traditional Surrogacy arrangements, which are referred to as "pre-planned adoption agreements", connects those contracts to State adoption law. Additionally, Florida law explicitly prohibits "homosexuals" from adopting. In 2004, this law was upheld in federal Court by the 11th Circuit Court of Appeals in the case of Lofton vs. Kearney.

Traditional Surrogacy is referred to as a "pre-planned adoption agreement" with a "voluntary mother" and requires court approval of the adoption. The most important distinctions between them is that, under pre-planned adoptions, the birth mother has 48 hours after the birth of the child to change her mind; the adoption must be approved by a court; and the Intended Parents do not have to be biologically related to the child.

In contrast, under a Gestational Surrogacy contract, the Surrogate must agree to relinquish her rights to the child upon birth; the Intended Mother must show that she cannot safely maintain a pregnancy or deliver a child; and at least one of the Intended Parents must be genetically related to the child. Both sets of laws require the Surrogate Mother to submit to medical evaluation; make the Surrogate the default parent if an Intended Parent who is expected to be a biological parent turns out not to be related to the child; limit the types of payment allowed; and require the Intended Parents to agree to accept any resulting child, regard-less of any impairment the child may have. Recruitment fees for Traditional Surrogates are prohibited.

Texas Surrogacy Law

Texas's law is modelled after Part 8 of the Uniform Parentage Act of 2002. A Gestational Surrogacy agree-ment must be validated by the court. It is against the law for the gestational mother to use her own eggs. To be a Surrogate Mother, she must have had at least one prior pregnancy and delivery. She will maintain control over all health-related decisions during the pregnancy. The Intended Mother must show that she is unable to carry a pregnancy or give birth. The Intended Parents must be married and must undergo a home study. There is a residence requirement of at least 90 days for either the gestational mother or the Intended Parents. An agreement that has not been validated is not enforceable, and parentage will be determined under the other parts of Texas's Uniform Parentage Act.

Virginia Surrogacy Law

Virginia requires pre-authorization of a surrogacy contract by a court. If the contract is approved, then the Intended Parents will be the legal parents. If the contract is voided, the Surrogate Mother and her husband, if any, will be named the legal parents and the Intended Parents will only be able to acquire parental rights through adoption. If the contract was never approved, then the Surrogate can file a consent form relinquishing rights to the child. But if she does not, the parental rights will vary based on whether either of the Intended Parents have a genetic relationship to the child. Depending on the circumstances, they may need to adopt in order to obtain parental rights. Notwithstanding all of the above, if the Surrogate is the genetic mother, she may terminate the contract within the first six months of pregnancy.

Virginia's requirements for court approval include: a home study; a finding that all parties meet the standards of fitness applicable to adoptive parents; the Surrogate must be married and have delivered at least one prior live birth; the parties must have undergone medical evaluations and counselling; the Intended Mother must be infertile or unable to bear a child; and at least one Intended Parent must be genetically related to the child. The Intended Parents must accept the child regardless of its health or appearance. The Surrogate retains sole responsibility for the clinical management of the pregnancy.

During the approval proceedings, the court must appoint counsel for the Surrogate and a guardian ad litem to represent the interests of any resulting children. The court's approval of assisted conception under the contract is effective for twelve months. Compensation beyond reasonable medical and ancillary costs is not allowed. Recruitment fees are punishable as a misdemeanour, and the parties may collect damages from the facilitator or agency. The law also provides for an allocation of costs when a non-validated contract is terminated under various circumstances.

The rest of the US

Here in brief, is a look through all the other States of the US.

Alabama The courts are generally favourable to surrogacy. However, statutory language exempts surrogacy from adoption laws and prohibitions on baby selling. In 1996, the Alabama Court of Civil Appeals gave implicit recognition to a surrogacy arrangement when it awarded custody of a child in a divorce case to the wife, who had no biological relationship to the child.

Alaska There is no law governing surrogacy at all in Alaska. The courts generally are favourable. In 1989 the Alaskan Supreme Court equated surrogacy with adoption, which seems a very positive way forward.

Arizona Arizona Statute forbids "Surrogate parent contracts", whether they are Traditional or Gestational. It provides that, in a surrogacy situation, the Surrogate is the legal mother of the child or children and, if she is married, her husband is the father. However, the Arizona Court of Appeals, a court of intermediate jurisdiction ruled in 1994 that the parentage presumption was rebuttable as to the Intended Mother.

Arkansas Arkansas law is highly favourable to surrogacy. There is a Statute declaring surrogacy agreements valid. The Statute details several types of parentage situations, and clearly establishes rights in each situation. More than once, the Arkansas Supreme Court has ruled in favour of Intended Parents.

Colorado There is no law governing surrogacy but the courts are generally favourable.

Connecticut There is no legal objection to surrogacy arrangements. With regard to Pre-Birth Orders, the Connecticut Supreme Court has ruled that the State Office of Vital Statistics of the Connecticut Department of Health must comply with such orders, even when the Intended Parents have no biological relationship.

Delaware Delaware case law indicates that all surrogacy agreements are contrary to public policy.

District of Columbia The District of Columbia forbids surrogacy. Those who violate the Statute may be fined up to $10,000, given a prison sentence of up to one year, or both.

Georgia There is no law governing surrogacy but the courts are generally favourable.

Hawaii There is no law governing surrogacy but the courts are generally favourable.

Idaho There is no law governing surrogacy but the courts are generally favourable.

Illinois Illinois has a Statute highly favourable to Gestational Surrogacy which governs the process from contract formation to the issuance of birth certificates. It applies to single parents who have furnished their own gametes (sperm or eggs), or heterosexual couples where at least one person who has furnished his or her own gametes. Illinois Law does not take into account a same-sex couple.

Indiana Under Indiana law, surrogacy contracts are, "void and unenforceable". Nevertheless, a few judges will grant Pre-Birth Orders.

Iowa The courts are generally favourable. Although Iowa has no surrogacy Statute, the Iowa Code exempts a "Surrogate Mother arrangement" from criminal provisions regarding the sale or purchase of human beings.

Kansas There is no law governing surrogacy, but two opinions of the Attorney General argued that surrogacy contracts are void as being against public policy.

Kentucky There is no law governing surrogacy. The Kentucky Supreme Court has indicated that surrogacy contracts are voidable by a party to the arrangement.

Louisiana A Louisiana Statute declares Traditional Surrogacy agreements to be void, unenforceable, and contrary to public policy. The Statute does not address Gestational Surrogacy. However, many courts are unfriendly towards Gestational Surrogacy.

Maine There is no law governing surrogacy but the courts are generally favourable.

Maryland There is no law governing surrogacy but the courts are generally favourable. However, an Attorney General's opinion from 2000 argued that compensated surrogacy contracts are illegal but did not oppose post-birth adoptions, indicating that the judge would have to consider the best interests of the child(ren).

Massachusetts There is no law governing surrogacy but the courts are generally favourable.

Michigan Michigan law forbids surrogacy. Individuals who enter into surrogacy arrangements may be fined up to $50,000 and imprisoned for up to five years.

Minnesota There is no law governing surrogacy but the courts are generally favourable.

Mississippi There is no law governing surrogacy but the courts are generally favourable.

Missouri There is no law governing surrogacy but the courts are generally favourable.

Montana There is no law governing surrogacy but the courts are generally favourable.

Nebraska Under Nebraska law "[a] Surrogate parenthood contract entered into shall be void and unenforceable". This provision applies to compensated surrogacy agreements in which the Surrogate "is compensated for bearing a child of a man who is not her husband".

Nevada Gestational surrogacy agreements are permitted only between legally married (heterosexual) couples.

New Hampshire New Hampshire law permits married heterosexual couples to become Intended Parents in Traditional or Gestational Surrogacy arrangements where one partner has furnished a gamete. The Statute does not appear to sanction Gestational Surrogacy arrangements in which a donor egg was used, and the legal position is unclear at the time of writing.

New Jersey New Jersey forbids Traditional Surrogacy but is friendly toward Gestational Surrogacy, remunerated or compassionate. Although the Attorney General opposes the granting of Pre-Birth Orders in Gestational Surrogacy cases involving an Egg Donor, the courts frequently issue such orders anyway.

New Mexico There is no law governing surrogacy but the courts are generally favourable.

North Carolina There is no law governing surrogacy but the courts are generally favourable.

North Dakota North Dakota law forbids Traditional Surrogacy but permits Gestational Surrogacy.

Ohio It is clear that the Ohio courts are deeply divided over the status of surrogacy. Accordingly, some judges are loathed to grant Pre-Birth Orders, but others are happy to do so.

Oklahoma Oklahoma has no law on surrogacy. An Attorney-General's opinion from 1983 that pre-dated the rise of Gestational Surrogacy declared that compensated surrogacy contracts violated the State's statutory prohibition on child trafficking.

Oregon The courts are generally surrogacy friendly and they will issue declarations of paternity.

Pennsylvania Pennsylvania has no law governing surrogacy. Some more conservative judges will not grant Pre-Birth Orders. The Pennsylvania adoption Statute provides for the post-birth adoption of a child born through surrogacy in the country of the Intended Parents' domicile.

Rhode Island There is no law governing surrogacy but the courts are generally favourable.

South Carolina There is no law governing surrogacy but the courts are generally favourable.

South Dakota There is no law governing surrogacy but the courts are generally favourable.

Tennessee Tennessee has a Statute that "expressly authorize(s) the Surrogate birth process". It defines surrogacy as comprising two situations: 1) Gestational Surrogacy where both Intended Parents furnish the gametes [egg and sperm]; and 2) Gestational Surrogacy where the Intended Father furnishes the sperm and the Surrogate relinquishes the child to him and his wife.

Utah Utah has a Statute permitting Gestational Surrogacy. It forbids Traditional Surrogacy and also does not allow the Surrogate's husband to act as the Sperm Donor. At least one Intended Parent must have furnished a gamete.

Vermont There is no law governing surrogacy but the courts are generally favourable.

Virginia Virginia permits surrogacy but has a Statute so complicated that the common practice for Virginia births is to file an action post-birth for amendment of the birth certificate.

Washington Washington Statutes permit uncompensated surrogacy arrangements but declare compensated ones void and unenforceable. Those involved in the latter are guilty of a gross misdemeanour.

West Virginia The courts are generally favourable. A Statute prohibiting human trafficking exempts fees and expenses in surrogacy arrangements.

Wisconsin The courts are generally favourable. A Statute governing the collection of vital statistics specifically directs the responsible authorities to place the names of the Intended Parents on the birth certificate once a court determines parental rights.

Wyoming There is no law governing surrogacy but the courts are generally favourable.

8. Surrogacy and the British Law

Background

Unfortunately for Intended Parents who are living in the UK, surrogacy arrangements are governed by the current guidelines operated by the Human Fertilisation and Embryology Authority (HFEA). These antiquated laws were originally created to protect the rights of Intended Parents conceiving with the help of Egg and/or Sperm Donors. (In retrospect, this makes no sense: if the biological addition of the other parent was being used, there was no need to make both parents legally regarded as the biological parent. It really should have been done on a case-by-case basis.)

With the introduction of this law, the rights of women who had conceived using a donor egg to be regarded as the legal mother were protected, along with the rights of a husband to be regarded as the legal father where donor sperm had been used. In the case of most surrogacies, though, the sperm is used of the Intended Father and not a Sperm Donor, which should be specific in the legislation instead of operating a blanket policy. Unfortunately, this has caused huge issues for Intended Parents who have had to turn to surrogacy to conceive. The process of Gestational Surrogacy was not thought of at the time, and so was not considered within the legislation.

As a result, at the time of birth the husband of a Surrogate is considered to be the baby's legal father even though he has no genetic link to the baby, and similarly the Surrogate is considered to be the baby's legal mother even when she has no genetic link either. This is why many people embarking on surrogacy in the UK are only interested in working with a Surrogate who is not married, as this means that the Intended Father, in most cases, can put his name down on the birth certificate from the start.

Now, with the recently introduced Section 30 of the Human Fertilisation and Embryology Act 1990, there is a positive way forward to rectifying this. The Intended Parents can, after the birth, apply for a "Parental Order" to reassign legal parenthood, provided that they meet various criteria designed to ensure that the arrangement in question is non-commercial and that everyone involved consents. This process is explained fully below.

In my opinion, though, further changes are still required, and in particular we need a more transparent policy on expenses. The Government needs to look at the full process of surrogacy, and the way it brings joy to those people who are blessed enough to be able to go through the process and have a positive outcome. They also need to look at the areas of the law that are encouraging exploitation of women around the world who live in areas where a few thousand pounds will have a life-changing effect.

We also need to review current maternity leave policy for parents who have a baby through surrogacy. Although this has been addressed within adoption law, other parents who have been unable to carry their own children are currently discriminated against. In short, our laws on surrogacy and maternity leave need to be dragged screaming and kicking into the twenty-first-century.

The importance of taking legal advice

The complexities of the law make it essential that Intending Parents take legal advice, both before and during the surrogacy process. However, over the years I have met many legal parasites who have grossly over-charged for very simple services in the process of creating a surrogacy arrangement. This does not need to be the case. Do not be frightened into accepting what a lawyer says because they are meant to be a great expert. In reality, given the relatively small number of cases that have been before UK courts to date, no one actually is.

However, there are some firms (listed in Appendix C) that have worked in the area of surrogacy law since it started to become popular in the mid 1990s. I would recommend that you give them a call before searching through the Yellow Pages or calling your usual family solicitor. Go to someone with relevant experience, and they will help you as much as they can.

One such firm is A City Law Firm LLP, who are based in the City of London. I asked one of the partners at the firm to write the following information and advice about the UK law, as I want you to have the best advice possible. I have added comments from my own perspective where relevant.

Introduction

Having a child is both an exciting and daunting prospect for any parent, but choosing to have a child via a surrogacy arrangement can be even more daunting due to the complex issues involved. Surrogacy arrangements are intricate and involve a number of different people, all with different and sometimes conflicting roles. Understanding the laws, risks, stages and process can be very stressful and confusing. The objective of this chapter is to break down the process and laws into digestible stages, so that we can simplify the issues in order for you to enjoy your journey and ultimately to remain in control at all times.

Choosing a Surrogate Mother is often full of emotive decisions, with some people using a family member or close friend and others using someone who is completely independent of them. Often people will utilise clinics and agencies to arrange the agreement, Surrogate and payments. These service providers can give you guidance and advice, and hopefully facilitate an efficient arrangement. However, they are not lawyers, and we cannot impress upon you enough the importance of understanding the responsibilities, legal requirements and procedures required for your personal situation. It is important that you take legal advice before, during and after the conception/birth, since being fully aware of your rights, the pitfalls and the procedures will promote a smooth and stress-free process for all involved.

Overview

The law in the UK has been evolving slowly. However, both the law and the related procedures still remain very complex and, compared with some other countries, very strict. Some countries, such as India, and some US States take a far more liberal approach, for example allowing Intended Parents to be named immediately on the birth certificates as the parents. Contracts will be considered binding and, in some countries commercial payments to the Surrogate Mother are permitted.

However, while it is immensely attractive to enter an arrangement abroad, if the Intended Parents are domiciled (a legal concept referring to where you consider your roots to be and intend to live permanently) in the UK, then English surrogacy law will apply irrespective of the international position. This can result in the Intended Parents having no status as the legal parents of the child in the UK, despite the foreign jurisdiction where the child was born acknowledging them as having full rights.

It has been considered by some that the law in England and Wales needs updating further to bring it in line with other jurisdictions. There have been some recent decisions in the High Court which have gradually begun to challenge this area of the law, and it will certainly be interesting to see how this continues to develop.

Stage 1: Understand the key issues prior to any arrangement

You need to understand the key factors that can prevent your surrogacy arrangement from being successful and prevent you from obtaining legal parental status. That way you remain in control and can overcome these hurdles. We have highlighted in brief below some of the key rules and thus the potential difficulties which can arise, but more detail on the same will be provided throughout this chapter.

First, you should note that although the terms of a surrogacy agreement may be considered by a UK Court if and when an application is made, it is not binding on the Court and it can choose to overrule any aspect. There are also strict deadlines that you need to be aware of, which are discussed in greater detail below. You should be aware at the outset that these are not negotiable, and the Court cannot extend them under any circumstances.

> • It is illegal in England and Wales for a surrogacy arrangement to be conducted for profit to the benefit of any party. Therefore, no more than "reasonable expenses" can be paid to the Surrogate Mother for the arrangement. If it is considered by the Court that more than this has been paid to the Surrogate Mother, then this could result in you being refused parental rights over the child even where you may have used a Surrogate abroad where it was legal to pay her. You need to

ensure that whoever is assisting with any arrangements understands these UK rules.

• Be aware there is a six-week cooling-off period in the UK. The Court will not make an order without the consent of the Surrogate Mother (and her husband/civil partner) being obtained following the birth, and this release cannot be signed until after a period of six weeks following the birth of the child. You should consult a lawyer in the chosen jurisdiction about whether such consent can be included in the surrogacy agreement.

• If you have the child abroad, it is important to be prepared so that you do not risk your child being denied entry by the UK Border Agency. The child may need leave to remain, or may need to apply for residency depending on your circumstances. Do not risk being denied access to the UK; get the facts before hand.

Barrie Drewitt-Barlow comments: "It is very important to recognise the six-week cooling-off period for your Surrogate. It is also important to remember the limit on the amount of expenses that you are able to pay your Surrogate. You should NOT be tempted to pay any more just to get the Surrogate that you want, because when it comes to the time of making the application for the Parental Rights Order, you will need to show how much in expenses you have spent."

Stage 2: Applying to Court following the birth to acquire full Parental Status and a UK Birth Certificate

What is a Parental Order?

In order for you, the Intended Parents, to obtain legal parental status in England and Wales, it is necessary to apply to the Courts for a Parental Order. Once a Parental Order is granted, a new UK birth certificate can be issued naming you both as the legal parents. This will confer all associated rights and responsibilities, as with any traditional parents. Sadly, until a Parental Order is granted — and irrespective of what the law says in the country where the surrogacy arrangement took place and where the child was born — English law will continue to regard the Surrogate Mother (and her husband/civil partner, if she has one) as the legal parent.

Why and when would you apply?

As the Intended Parents you would apply for a Parental Order in order to obtain legal status and recognition as the parents of the child. The application must be made to the UK Court within six months of the child's birth. You must bear in mind that the consent of the

Surrogate Mother will not be considered valid by the Court until the 'cooling-off' period of six weeks from the child's birth has elapsed. However, the six-month period of time must be adhered to as there is no ability to extend it. If you miss it, your application will be denied.

Who can apply?

Previously, the law in England and Wales only permitted married couples to apply for a Parental Order. The law has recently changed, and from 6 April 2010 the Human Fertilisation and Embryology Act 2008 extended the right to apply for Parental Orders to unmarried couples. This includes couples who are in a same-sex relationship, whether in a civil partnership or co-habiting. The law did not extend this right to single persons.

The Criteria for applying for a Parental Order

As mentioned above, the application for a Parental Order is regulated by very strict conditions which must be met in order for the Court to grant the Order. The criteria to be met are as follows:

The Application

• The application must be made within six months of the birth of the child; and

• The Court will issue a form which the Surrogate (and her husband/civil partner) must sign six weeks after the birth to show their consent.

The Applicants (the Intended Parents):

• Must be at least 18 years old.

• Must be married, civil partners or co-habiting in an enduring relationship.

• At least one of the Intended Parents must be the biological parent.

• At the time of the application and at the time the Order is made, at least one Intended Parent must be domiciled in the UK. (For these purposes, domiciled means where you consider your roots are and live permanently.)

The Surrogacy Arrangement

• The child must live with the Intended Parents/applicants at the time of the application and at the time the order is made.

• The child must be born to a Surrogate as a result of conception taking place through artificial insemination.

• No more than reasonable expenses must have been paid to the Surrogate Mother. The Court will consider this carefully and will decide what amounts to a reasonable expense on a case-by-case basis. This will be considered further below, but as already mentioned this can lead to applications being rejected where the courts may view the arrangement to be commercial.

• The Surrogate and her husband/civil partner have consented to the application. (Any husband or civil partner will automatically be deemed to be the father or other parent of the child). This consent must be given at least six weeks after the birth.

Stage 3: The Court Process

The application is made and heard in the Family Proceedings Court (Magistrates Court). As mentioned above, the Court will issue an acknowledgement form to you requesting the specific consent of the Surrogate and her partner to the Order. You will therefore need to send this to them and later return it to the Court.

At the first hearing, the Court will usually arrange for a Parental Order Reporter to prepare a report and timetable any other directions it may require in order to assist in making a decision. The Reporter effectively acts as the eyes and ears of the Court, undertaking enquiries and investigations into the circumstances of the case, and reports to the Court their findings. In an application for a Parental Order, their task is to report to the Court on whether the conditions/criteria for applying for a Parental Order set out above are met, and also to confirm that it is in the child's welfare and best interests to make the order. The Court will then have regard to this report when considering making its decision. Usually the officer will wish to meet with both of you and, where feasible, the Surrogate and any legal partner too. The time it takes to prepare this report will depend on how busy the Reporters in the local area are, and it could take anything from three to six months.

The Court may well also direct that each party to the application file a personal statement setting out their personal position. In order to ensure that your position is clearly and succinctly put to the Reporter, it is advisable to have your lawyers prepare detailed statements on behalf of you and your partner, and where possible for the Surrogate Mother, before issuing the Parental Order application. This will provide the Reporter with the background information that they need to understand everyone's intentions, personal circumstances and objectives from the start, which will help to support your application.

The Court will then hold a second hearing where it will consider the report of the Reporter and any other evidence presented. On the basis that there are no issues arising as a result of the report, that no one contests the application and the Court is satisfied, the Parental Order should be granted. However, if there are complications then the case may well be transferred to the County Court or the High Court. Due to their complexity, cases involving international surrogacy arrangements are usually transferred automatically to the High Court. Once the Parental Order has been issued, you can then apply immediately for a new UK birth certificate with both your names shown as the legal parents.

Reasonable expenses:
What are these?

As stated above, surrogacy arrangements taking place in England and Wales are heavily regulated. A surrogacy arrangement is not illegal in itself. However, it is illegal for the surrogacy to take place as a commercial arrangement, or to advertise that you are looking for or are willing to act as a Surrogate. If you are applying for a Parental Order and your agreement in the US, for example, shows that you paid a fee for the Surrogate's services rather than just expenses, the Court can deny your application here in the UK.

Barrie Drewitt-Barlow comments: "The agreement that you set up with a US-based Surrogate should mention a 'base fee'. This base fee should be no higher than the normal amount. However, in the UK, an agreement is NOT a legally binding agreement that can be relied upon in a UK court, so it need not be presented to the court. With this in mind, we would suggest that disclosure of expenses should be made by separate documentation. This should be either a typed or a handwritten account of what you have spent on expenses for the Surrogate during her pregnancy. This does not need to include your travel, legal fees, medical fees at fertility clinics etc, only what money has changed hands between you and your Surrogate since the time of the pregnancy confirmation."

So, what 'reasonable expenses' are permitted?. There is no set budget, only an array of guidance indicators and case law that we can use to advise you. Expenses are however, just that — costs incurred by the Surrogate Mother as a direct result of the pregnancy. In exceptional cases, where there have been difficulties with the pregnancy and additional medical costs have been incurred, or there has been a loss of income, this could push the expenses above what was anticipated, which if evidenced is acceptable.

Basically, evidencing reasonable expenses to a court will require receipts, cheques, invoices and any other means by which you are able to show what the monies have been spent on, and, more importantly that these are legitimate expenses for the pregnancy. The court will take an overall picture of the case. However, anything not documented by an invoice or receipt may be regarded as profit and will not be accepted, and can lead to the arrangement being deemed to be commercial. The Court is keen to emphasise that this is done on a case-by-case basis.

On an application for a Parental Order, the Court will consider the expenses that have been paid. If the Court deems that more than reasonable expenses have been paid it may deny you the Parental Order, or it may raise further questions and difficulties before the Order is made.

Barrie Drewitt-Barlow comments: "it is important to note that the courts are working on the application that YOU submit. Therefore, it is also important to note that they work with the figures YOU give them. In the UK, we would recommend a limit of between £12-15,000."

Surrogacy Agreements

Surrogacy agreements are documents which are prepared as a form of contract between you, the Intended Parents, and the Surrogate Mother (and, if applicable, her partner). Such documents can set out the specific terms of the arrangements, such as the clinic to be used, the amount of expenses payable, the documents that they are required to sign (such as the six-week release form) etc. In some countries these documents are legally binding on the parties. However under the law of England and Wales, although Surrogacy Agreements can be referred to and persuasive to a Court, they are not binding on them.

Therefore, in short, whilst the parties may have entered into a 'contract' as to the terms of their arrangement, a Court is not bound by the contents of the document and can make a very different decision to that which is set out as the intentions of the parties within the surrogacy agreement. That said, however, the courts may well have regard to the agreement's contents in terms of it providing a background to the matter. As such, an agreement can be persuasive and help the Court understand the intentions of all parties. Ultimately, though, any decision made by the Court will not be based on the contents of the surrogacy agreement, but on what the Court deems to be in the best interests of the child.

It is worth noting that it is a criminal offence for any solicitor to draft the terms of a surrogacy agreement or negotiate on your behalf. We can only advise you on the effect and meaning of the contents and provide general guidance as to the considerations you should have.

Barrie Drewitt-Barlow comments: "The British Surrogacy Centre can help you with drafting your agreements with your potential Surrogate and Egg Donor. After years of experience advising on UK and US contracts/agreements, the BSC have become experts in assessing individual requirements and putting them into a document that can be set before the Court to evidence what the initial agreement was for all parties. As stated above, the Court does not legally have to take the content of the agreement into account when deciding a case. However, we feel that it is important to be able to show the Court the intention of all parties in writing."

Consent of the Surrogate Mother

One difficulty that can arise, and has indeed arisen in the past, is where the Surrogate Mother refuses to consent to give up the child to the Intended Parents. As already mentioned, she needs to provide her consent six weeks after the birth, and if she refuses to give consent then your application for a Parental Order may well be denied. Hopefully, such situations will remain few and far between. However, if an application is made to the courts, the Court will make a decision based on what it deems to be in the best interests of the child. As above, it will not bound by the terms of any surrogacy agreement, although it may be supportive of your intentions at the outset.

International surrogacy arrangements

Given that it is not permitted for a surrogacy arrangement to be a commercial arrangement in the UK, it is becoming more common for Intended Parents to travel abroad where such arrangements are permitted and the law in that jurisdiction offers greater protection to them. However, as stated previously, upon returning to the jurisdiction of England and Wales, English law will take precedence over the legal provisions of a foreign jurisdiction. A surprising number of people enter into a surrogacy arrangement without obtaining any advice in respect of both their legal position as parents and, if the surrogacy is taking place abroad, in respect of the immigration status of the child.

In many foreign jurisdictions, a surrogacy agreement is legally binding. However, as stated above, this is not the case in England, and as such a Court can overrule the terms of that agreement. Also, in some jurisdictions it is possible for the Intended Parents to be automatically named on the birth certificate as the parents, or to obtain an order from the Court granting the

Intended Parents legal status prior to the birth of the child. However, the law in England and Wales can differ dramatically from these provisions, and may not recognise the Intended Parents as being the parents despite the recognition given to them abroad. This can lead to a child being effectively parentless and stateless if you remain resident in the UK with your child.

Once the Intended Parents have returned to the UK with the child, the application for a Parental Order is the same as set out above, and the same criteria need to be met. However, it is essential that advice specific to the circumstances of your case is taken both in England and abroad in relation to parental status and immigration/citizenship matters. We have set out below the main difficulties that can arise following a surrogacy arrangement involving an international element.

Barrie Drewitt-Barlow comments: "There has not been any case to date where the UK Home Office has refused entry to a child born through surrogacy and has asked the Intended Parents to remove that child from the UK. In fact, the UK Home office has worked diligently over the past few years to recognise that people are going abroad to find options to becoming parents because of the strict, archaic laws that we have in Britain. However, it is still important to operate strictly within the law. As well as taking advice overseas, professional legal representation should ALWAYS be sought once you arrive back in the UK to make sure that all your paperwork is handled in the correct manner."

Reasonable expenses for a foreign Surrogate

One of the common pitfalls faced by parents returning with a child following an international surrogacy arrangement is that the arrangement has clearly been a commercial arrangement, as more than reasonable expenses appear to have been paid to the Surrogate Mother. A recent decision made in the High Court in Re L 2010 specifically addressed these difficulties, and has made a fundamental change in the way that Courts will now view the issue of "reasonable expenses".

The issue of what constituted a reasonable expense has always been unclear and dealt with on a case-by-case basis, and this still remains the case. However in the case concerned, Mr Justice Hedley ruled that, even where more than reasonable expenses have been paid, the Court must have the child's welfare as its paramount concern. It therefore should not withhold the making of a Parental Order if it is in the child's best interests to grant one — i.e. that it would cause more harm to the child if the Order were not made. This has been further affirmed in the recent case of Re IJ 2011, where it was ordered that, despite a higher level of expenses being paid than would usually be accepted in England and Wales, it was considered in the best interests of the child to make the Parental Order.

Barrie Drewitt-Barlow comments: "We have to look at this positive step forward by these two courts as the developing future of the legal system when it comes to this new area of law. With this in mind, it is of paramount importance that everything is done by the book and that you have proper legal advice throughout the process. It is also vital that you can show the court the intentions of all parties throughout the process by keeping proper accounts of what you have spent during your surrogacy."

Immigration issues that can arise

If the surrogacy arrangement takes place abroad, a factor of paramount concern is whether the parents will be able to bring the child back to the UK. Immigration law and issues of citizenship are incredibly complicated, and are very much determined by each cases' particular circumstance. On the basis that you will be considered the legal parent of the child for the purposes of satisfying English legislation and you are a British citizen, then the child will normally be entitled to British Citizenship at birth. However, if English law does not consider and treat either Intended Parent as the legal parent, then the law may not treat your child as being British at birth. If the child is not entitled to British citizenship at birth, then the child may have no automatic right to enter the UK. It may then be necessary to apply for a discretionary grant of citizenship and/or entry clearance.

Serious difficulties can arise if the Surrogate Mother is married or in a civil partnership, as even if the Intended Father is the biological father, the law will recognise the Surrogate's husband/partner as the parent despite them having no biological link. In order to avoid the above complexities, it may be easier to use a Surrogate who is single. However, some Intended

Parents have objections to this, and specifically wish for the Surrogate to be married or in a civil partnership. If this is the case, it is essential that the husband/partner is fully willing to give their consent to the Parental Order at the time that the application is made, and we recommend bringing them into the surrogacy agreement where possible.

It is essential that you seek specialist immigration advice prior to entering any surrogacy arrangement involving a foreign jurisdiction. This will ensure that both yours and the child's position is protected and a smooth return to the UK following the birth of the child.

Advice in the foreign jurisdiction

If the surrogacy arrangement is taking place abroad, it is of course important to obtain detailed legal advice from an expert in any foreign jurisdiction involved to ensure that the legal position there is fully understood. It should be noted that, while agencies can be helpful, they may provide simplistic advice which may not adequately or comprehensively address your particular circumstances, so be armed with UK and applicable jurisdictional advice from a qualified lawyer.

Barrie Drewitt-Barlow comments: "Your agency should be able to provide general advice on the legal aspects of a surrogacy in the country where it is based. If they cannot, then ask them to get the information for you; after all, that's why you're paying fees. But please remember that, while some agencies are owned by lawyers, not all are. In any case, it is VERY important to take independent legal advice away from the agency that you are working with, because your best interests may be in conflict with theirs. Your independent legal team will only be working for you."

Common Questions

When can I apply for a Parental Order and how long will it take?

Any application for a Parental Order must be made within six months of the birth and there is no ability to extend this time frame. You must bear in mind the six-week cooling-off period for the valid consent of the Surrogate Mother. How long it will take to conclude the application will depend on the Court and the Parental Order Reporter. Generally speaking, you will be looking at a time period of four to six months.

Do we need a Parental Order?

This is a frequently asked question, given the daunting prospect of making an application to the Courts — especially given the strict conditions to be met, and not least the time and expense which can be incurred. The legal position and implications of not applying for a Parental Order depends on the legal status of the Intended Parents.

If the Intended Father is recognised as the legal father of the child, then he is legally permitted to care for his child. (This is on the basis that the birth is registered in the UK and his name is on the birth certificate.) The other Intended Parent, either the Intended Mother or non-biological father, will remain insecure. This could lead to potential difficulties in the future, such as if the Intended Parents were to separate or the Intended Father were to die.

If neither Intended Parent is recognised as the legal parent of the child (when the surrogacy has taken place abroad), then neither Intended Parent will have the authority or legal right to care for the child. This includes the right to make any decision in respect of the child's welfare, such as consent to medical treatment. This can cause difficulties, especially where it is not practical to obtain the Surrogate's involvement on a day-to-day basis.

It is also worth bearing in mind that it is a criminal offence to care for a child if you have no legal right to do so. If you do not have a Parental Order or legal right to look after your child, it may be necessary for any authorities who you come into contact with to involve social services.

Barrie Drewitt-Barlow comments: "However, realistically, this is happening all the time. Surrogacy arrangements that have and are happening around the world with UK-based parents have worked extremely well for those people who have not applied for the Parental Orders. I have five children, all born in the US and to two different Surrogate Mothers, both of whom were married at the time of the birth. My partner and I do NOT have a UK Parental Order. The current restriction that says you cannot apply for the Parental Order before six weeks old and after the cut-off period of six months has meant that it is impossible for us to apply for it. In any case, we feel that the orders from the US courts give us enough rights and we are happy to stick with this. It is however my recommendation that if you can apply for the Parental Order in the UK, then you should do it. It will give you that extra legal right that is well worth having."

If I can't get or do not wish to get a Parental Order, what other options do I have?

If you decide not to proceed with a Parental Order application or it is refused, then there are alternative options available to you in order to secure your position as parents. These include making an application to the Court for Adoption, a Residence Order or a Special Guardianship Order. However, none of these provide you with the status or recognition that a Parental Order would in terms of being recognised as birth parents.

If you apply for an Adoption Order, this can be a slow and invasive procedure, with the Courts undertaking a detailed investigation into your circumstances. If an Adoption Order is granted, you will then be issued with an adoption certificate (rather than a new birth certificate). This will effectively mean that you are able to make all the decisions in relation to the child and they will be treated as your own. It will extinguish the Surrogate parents' rights over the child.

A Special Guardianship Order, if made, will enable you to have Parental Responsibility (providing you with the ability to make the day-to-day decisions in the child's life). However, they will not extinguish the Surrogate parents' rights, with them still being considered the legal parents of the child.

A Residence Order is an order that the child must live with you, and this will provide you with Parental Responsibility which enables you to make the day-to-day decisions in respect of the child's life. However, the Surrogate would still, for the purposes of English law, be considered the legal parent.

Conclusion

It is hoped that the above has provided a useful insight into the legal difficulties that can be faced by those entering into a surrogacy arrangement and, more importantly, how those difficulties can be addressed.

The law in England, Wales, Scotland and NI is very strict for those entering into surrogacy arrangements and this has been for policy reasons, the main one being that it is illegal for an arrangement to be for commercial profit. This has led to our legal system being far stricter than others and has created a direct conflict in laws, especially given globalisation and the ease of travelling leading to couples choosing to go abroad. The law has evolved over the last few years, with decisions being made by the courts that put the child's best interests as the paramount consideration when making a Parental Order. This is a vitally important step as, for all concerned, the child's welfare and well-being is the goal that all parties are trying to achieve. The law is still developing and being tested, though, so it will certainly be interesting to see how, as more cases are presented to the Courts, the law continues to develop.

Surrogacy arrangements are never going to be an easy way to have a family. However, if all parties are in agreement, each respective position is understood, and the appropriate steps are taken to ensure they are protected, this will assist in making your dream of having a family a smoother journey for all concerned.

Appendix A: Common Terms and Acronyms

Terms

Surrogate Mother or Surrogate Carrier The woman who carries the child for someone else.

Gestational Surrogate Mother or Gestational Carrier A woman who goes through IVF to become pregnant as a Surrogate Mother using an egg from another woman who may be the Intended Mother or an Egg Donor. The baby or babies she carries have no biological link to her whatsoever.

Traditional Surrogate Mother or Traditional Carrier A woman who goes through Artificial Insemination with the sperm of the Intended Father or a donor to become pregnant as a Surrogate Mother. The baby or babies she carries are biologically her own children. She will sign over the legal rights to these children at birth.

Egg Donor The woman who, in some surrogacy arrangements, donates her own eggs (ova) to the process. A woman does not need to be involved in surrogacy to be termed an Egg Donor.

Intended Parents (IPs) The parents of the baby or babies carried by the Surrogate Mother. These are the parents the surrogacy is intended for. At least one of the Intended Parents may be biologically related to the Surrogate babies.

Intended Mother The mother of the baby the Surrogate is carrying. She may or may not be a biological relative of the child.

Intended Father The father of the baby the Surrogate is carrying. He may or may not be a biological relative of the child.

Intended Fathers When plural, Intended Fathers usually refers to a set of Intended Parents that are gay. Thus, there are two Intended Fathers instead of just one.

Acronyms

The following surrogacy acronyms are comprised of terms directly related to Surrogate Motherhood, and which are commonly used in discussions online. There are many other definitions of surrogacy acronyms that are used on message boards and in blogs, but this covers the industry specific ones.

SM Surrogate Mother

GS Gestational Surrogate Mother or Gestational Carrier

TS Traditional Surrogate Mother or Traditional Carrier

ED Egg Donor

IP or IPs Intended Parent(s)

IM Intended Mother

IF Intended Father

IFs Intended Fathers

2ww The Two Week Wait (this is the time after a transfer that the Surrogate and Intended Parents wait before finding out if the transfer was successful).

AI Artificial Insemination

BCP Birth Control Pills

BFN Big Fat Negative

BFP Big Fat Positive

CD Cycle Day

D & C Dilation & Curettage

ET Embryo Transfer

FET Frozen Embryo Transfer

HPT Home Pregnancy Test

IVF In Vitro Fertilization

PG Pregnant

PIO Progesterone in Oil

PIP Previous (or potential) Intended Parents

PIF Previous (or potential) Intended Father

POAS Pee on a Stick (when taking a home pregnancy test)

RE Reproductive Endocrinologist

STD Sexually Transmitted Disease

TTC Trying to Conceive

US Ultrasound

Appendix B:
Sex Selection

Wikipedia describes sex selection as "the attempt to control the sex of the offspring to achieve a desired sex". In many cultures, many women do certain things, eat certain things and pray to their gods for a particular gender of child to be born. Sex selection is also known as "Family Balancing", and has been marketed as a money back guarantee to couples desiring a particular sex of child. Sex selection can be accomplished in several ways.

Gradient Method

The gradient method is one of the simplest forms of sex selection technology. Sperm from the father is placed in a rapidly spinning machine called a centrifuge. As it spins, this machine helps to separate sperm with Y-chromosomes from those with X-chromosomes, which are heavier due to having more genetic material. Some people argue that the gradient method is associated with poorer success rates, but it is also less expensive than other sex selection options which is why a lot of people choose this option.

Flow Cytometry

Another sperm-sorting technique is Flow Cytometry. This method uses fluorescent dye to highlight sperm that carry X chromosomes by adhering to genetic material within the sperm. Because X-bearing sperm contain more genetic material, these sperm pick up more dye than the Y-bearing sperm. A laser machine is then used to separate the two types of sperm. The sperm with the appropriate chromosomes are then used in IUI or IVF. Success rates with Flow Cytometry are high: you have a 60% to 70% of conceiving a child of the desired gender.

Pre-implantation Genetic Diagnosis (PGD)

Although this method is complex, as it involves DNA analysis of a cell from an embryo, it is said to be the most successful of all the methods available when it comes to gender selection. Three or four days following fertilisation using IVF, one cell from each dividing embryo is removed and analyzed for DNA and other genetic material. Once the sex of the embryos are determined, only those embryos of the desired sex are implanted into the mother's uterus through IVF. PGD is highly successful, giving you a 99% chance of having a child of the desired gender.

Costs of Sex Selection

Sex selection isn't cheap, but couples are still opting for this method more frequently now. The average cost is anywhere between $600-$3500.

Ethical and Legal Concerns

Sex selection is certainly a topic that creates a lot of debate in countries all over the world. There are those people who would argue that sex selection perpetuates sexual discrimination and stereotyping. Sex selection also impacts negatively on the ratio of male to female births in countries such as India, where it is estimated that some 5000 females are aborted each week, even late on into the pregnancy. This is expected to cause growing difficulties in the future as large numbers of men will be unable to find partners, and is already resulting in the kidnapping of girls and women.

Despite this, social sex selection is actually illegal in India, and to ensure this prenatal determination of sex through ultrasound is also illegal. Similarly sex selection is officially prohibited in China, but the Chinese government is aware that the practice is widespread, especially in rural areas of China.

Some countries, such as the UK, severely restrict access to PGD technology in particular. The HFEA (Human Fertilisation and Embryo Authority) have banned sex selection in the UK unless you can show a serious gender-linked disorder in the family, such as haemophilia or Duchenne's Muscular Dystrophy which only affects boys. There are many devastating genetic disorders that can only be passed on to children of one particular sex. With this in mind, the HFEA say that they are happy to consider UK couples for sex selection procedures under these circumstances.

Some people feel that, if we allow sex selection now, where will it stop? Will we try to select other characteristics of our children, including hair colour, eye colour, and intelligence level? It is also the case that, by pre-selecting embryos by gender, the chances of achieving a successful pregnancy are reduced. In some cases, all of the embryos resulting from an IVF cycle may be of one gender, or the best quality embryos may not be of the desired gender. You need to think very carefully before opting for any of these processes, but don't rule it out if it is something you feel strongly about.

If you do opt for sex selection, it is available at most fertility clinics throughout the United States. There currently is no body that governs sex selection procedures, and fertility clinics may offer it at their own discretion. Hundreds of couples each year therefore travel to the US for sex selection of embryos, usually because they already have two or more children of one gender and none of the other. This is normally referred to as fertility tourism. The HFEA are aware that couples from the UK travel abroad to have sex selection procedures carried out, but they are unable to do anything about it as it falls outside of their jurisdiction.

Appendix C:
Further Sources of
Information and Support

"When we were told by our IVF specialist that he would not be happy to try another IVF cycle with Sandra, we just thought that we would never have children. However, he mentioned that he had seen a news report on the BBC that a new surrogacy centre was opening in Essex, and that maybe we should contact them about help through the surrogacy process. We got in contact with the British Surrogacy Centre and arranged a meeting at their Essex Site. After the initial meeting things started to move very quickly, and before you knew it we had a meeting with a potential Surrogate and Egg Donor. That was six months ago and we are now pregnant with twin girls! The best decision we have ever made."

Jason and Sandra, Manchester, UK

Fertility Specialists in the UK & US

Issues to be aware of when deciding on a clinic

I have, over the past 14 years, worked with many fertility clinics, both as a patient and as a referral source. There are countless clinics around the UK, and the number is growing all the time.

It's hard for anyone going through infertility to decide on where to go for treatment. The important thing is that you feel comfortable in terms of the treatment you are getting from the clinic, and also with the treatment that your Surrogate will receive from them. I have seen cases where medical directors of facilities have been incredibly rude to both the Intended Parents and the Surrogate (or Egg Donor), and have questioned the motives of the Surrogate. I find this behaviour very hard to understand from so-called professionals.

The moment that you feel uncomfortable with your fertility clinic, and especially with the treating consultant, it's time to go! Do not feel that they are your last hope, because they are not. There will be another hundred clinics that will treat you better, and they will also do a better job for you because they will want to make your dreams come true. I have talked with many couples over the years who say that they can't understand why they have gone through 5-8 IVF cycles and transfers and still cannot get pregnant. Then they mention that their consultant always seemed edgy around them, or short with them when answering questions.

The fact is that not every consultant wants your cycle

to work, and the quicker you identify this, the better off you will be. Personally, I can never understand how a consultant or a clinic can continue to take your money and not deliver a positive end result. Before you decide on the clinic to use, make sure that they have arrangements in place to help you if you do not achieve a pregnancy during the first couple of attempts, such as discounts on further cycles. So you might pay 100% the first time, 50% for the second, 30% for the third etc. Unfortunately, all too often "unexplained infertility" is used as a get-out clause. Why is it unexplained? Because they haven't found the reason. Often this is something that should have been identified early on, and saved you thousands of pounds as well as a lot of grief into the process.

Some people have asked me in the past about the incentive for a consultant to make sure that they achieve a positive result during the first cycle, because if the cycle fails, the consultant gets paid all over again. Well, there is no doubt that, around the world, some consultants are better than others at achieving positive results earlier on. It is your job to make sure that you seek out these consultants and do your homework. Use internet searches and chat forums; people are VERY happy to to shout about the good and bad experiences they have had.

If you cannot find a thread on the internet about a particular clinic, then you need to start one. Ask the question, "What do you know about ... clinic, and what experiences have you had there?" Trust me, people will tell you, warts and all. At the British Surrogacy Centre, we are updating our lists all the time in terms of who and where we recommend to go to for services. The lists change because employees at a facility, or the service providers operating a facility, change, and when they do, sometimes so does the standard of service. Please keep checking the web site for up to date information: www.britishsurrogacycentre.com

However, we can recommend the following with confidence:

Birmingham Women's Fertility Centre
Mindelsohn Way
Edgbaston
Birmingham B15 2TG
+ 44 (0)121 627 2700

Birmingham Women's Fertility Centre has been providing exceptional care to couples and individuals experiencing fertility problems for over 30 years. They are an expert team employing a holistic approach to your treatment. They are the only NHS-based specialist Fertility Unit in Birmingham licensed to provide a full range of services from diagnosis of infertility; to specialist fertility surgery; assisted conception treatment; and pre-implantation genetic diagnosis (PGD).

Bourn Hall Clinic
Charter Court
Newcomen Way
Colchester
Essex CO4 9YA
Tel: + 44 (0)1206 844454
Contact: Sarah Pallett.

Bourn Hall is a leading fertility clinic. There is no doubt that, over the past 30 years, they have been pioneers in the developing areas of IVF. I am happy to recommend the Colchester clinic as I have experience of working with some of the team there on surrogacy cases. Again, please do check the website for updates.

California Fertility Partners
11818 Wilshire Blvd, Suite 300
Los Angeles,
CA 90025
Dr Guy Ringler
Gringler@aol.com
Tel: 310-828-4008

I have had personal experience of working with this clinic for well over a decade. California Fertility Partners is a Los Angeles clinic dedicated to infertility testing and fertility treatments. With over 30 years experience in both fertility research and clinical practice, the Los Angeles center is recognized as one of the country's premier practices for fertility care. Dr Guy Ringler is seen by many as THE leading US fertility clinician.

The London Women's Clinic
113 - 115 Harley Street
London W1G 6AP UK
Tel: +44 (0)20 7563 4309
info@londonwomensclinic.com

Established 1985 in Harley Street, The London Women's Clinic pioneered many of the fertility treatments now considered routine with assisted conception. This clinic is happy to work with surrogacy and Sperm Donors, but as of June 2011 had a long waiting time for egg dona-tion services of 12-18 months. Well worth a telephone call to though.

CARE Manchester
108 -112 Daisy Bank Road
Victoria Park
Manchester M14 5QH.
+44 (0)161 249 3040
+44 (0)161 224 4283
info@carefertility.com

Manchester Fertility Services Ltd
Bridgewater Hospital
120 Princess Road, Manchester M15 5AT
+44 (0)161 227 0010
Fax: +44 (0)161 227 0011
info@manchesterfertility.com

The Lister Fertility Clinic
The Lister Hospital
Chelsea Bridge Road
London SW1W 8RH
+44 (0)20 7730 5932

Legal Services

Legal issues will be of huge concern throughout your surrogacy journey. You should make sure that, legally, every aspect of your journey has a legal eye watching over it. In the UK, a lawyer is limited in the services that s/he can provide to you regarding your surrogacy, but they are able to help with issues concerning immigration and Parental Orders etc. However, I have worked with and recommended several firms over the years that I no longer refer clients to. This is mainly because they got greedy and started to charge ridiculous amounts of money for services that really should not cost so much.

Several firms will give you a set price for a service package now, rather than billing you at an hourly rate. It is a good idea to get this sorted out at the beginning of negotiations with the firm, because you do not want to be hit with a huge bill at the end of the process. Agree an upfront amount, so that whatever hours the firm work on your case, the end figure is never going to change. Again, remember, the law firm is not God! They are there to assist you in getting through the process legally to the end result of you arriving home with your baby. If they are not doing a good enough job, get rid of them and work with someone who will give you a better service.

A City Law Firm
2 Devonshire Square
London EC2M 4UJ
+44 (0)20 7426 0382
Fax: +44 (0)20 7426 0180
Email: enquiries@acitylawfirm.com
Contact: Karen Holden

This is a recently established firm, but our preferred partner of choice at the time of writing (June 2011). This firm offers a much lower rate than any other UK practice at this time for dealing with the legal issues involved in surrogacy. For the past year, we have worked closely with this firm to establish a price list that reflects the already burdensome amounts of money that you have spent or are about to spend. They are a caring, compassionate firm that work with a cross-section of clients and will work with you in getting all the necessary paperwork sorted out for your return into the UK with your baby(ies).

Reproductive Law Center, Inc.
8419 La Mesa Blvd., Suite C
La Mesa,
CA 91942
Email: info@rlcsd.com
Tel: (619) 464-6640
Contact: Tom Pinkerton

Reproductive Law Center is committed to providing you and your family with extraordinary legal support in all aspects of family formation, whether you reside in the United States or are travelling to the United States from another country. They also provide a free initial consultation to set you on the right path. I have personally worked with Tom Pinkerton for over a decade and can confirm that he is THE leading legal expert in family formations anywhere in the US. Tom was instrumental in obtaining my own judgements in 1998, 2003 and again in 2010. Over the years he has worked on thousands of surrogacy cases.

Dawson Cornwell
15 Red Lion Square
London
England
+44 (0)20 7242 2556
mail@dawsoncornwell.com
Contact: Anne-Marie Hutchins

I highly recommend Anne-Marie Hutchins at Dawson Cornwell for advice on international surrogacy arrangements. She has a wealth of knowledge in the area and has worked with some high-profile cases over the years. Anne-Marie advises in respect of complex domestic and international adoption applications and legal issues arising from the creation and implementation of surrogacy arrangements and The Human Fertilisation and Embryology Act 2008. This is a high-end firm, and as such expect to pay high fees for the services. Certainly worth having a chat to though, to make sure you have everything covered.

Natalie Gamble
19 Glasshouse Studios
Fryern Court Roa,
Burgate
Nr Salisbury
SP6 1QX
+44 (0)844 357 1603
natalie@nataliegambleassociates.com

This company claims to be the only specialist fertility and parenting law firm in the UK devoted exclusively to UK and international surrogacy, donor conception and co-parenting, fertility treatment and embryo law, and parenting involving same-sex parents and other non-traditional families. I have no experience of them whatsoever apart from sharing some time with one of the firm's lawyers on Woman's Hour with Jenni Murray. As more information becomes available on each of these firms, I will be updating the website links and comments.

Information and Advice

The British Surrogacy centre (USA)
Suite 110
West Park Executive
672 West 11th Street
Tracy, CA 95376
001 209 229 7745
Email: DonnaCalabrese@Britishsurrogacycentre.com

The team behind BSC, including the author of this book, have been involved in surrogacy and egg donation since 1994. Over half of our team members have been through the process of surrogacy and egg donation themselves. We are dedicated to building the families of the future and to giving ordinary people the chance to have a family of their own. Our aim is to help you through the process of your surrogacy, Egg Donor, sperm donation or co-parenting arrangement. Please note that we do NOT advertise for Surrogates or Egg Donors in Europe, they find us and register with us freely.

To Hatch
07956 363030
Camille@to-hatch.co.uk
www.to-hatch.co.uk
Contact: Camille Strachan

This charity exists to provide key information on fertility treatments, clinics, services and products. It is a small yet powerful hub of knowledge with the help of and supporting data from the NHS and the HFEA.

Sperm Banks / Providers

Pride Angel http://www.prideangel.com/

Pride Angel is a UK limited company founded by professional scientists Erika and Karen. With personal experience of donor conception and raising children within a lesbian relationship, together they are committed to helping single, lesbian, gay and infertile couples become parents through donor conception and co-parenting. Pride Angel is dedicated to matching Sperm Donors, egg donors and co-parents worldwide.

European Sperm Bank ApS
Falkoner Allé 63, 2 floor
2000 Frederiksberg
Copenhagen
Denmark
+45 38343600

European Sperm Bank USA
4915 25th Avenue NE, Suite 204
Seattle
WA 98105
1-800-709 1223
info@europeanspermbankusa.com

Cryos International - Denmark ApS
Vesterbro Torv 1-3, 5th floor
DK-8000 Aarhus C.
Denmark
+45 86760699
dk@cryosinternational.com

References

Thailand

New Draft Law to Regulate Surrogacy in Thailand by Melanie Adams, 24 June 2010, Thai Law Forum.

India

Surrogacy Arrangements: Comparative Dimensions and Prospective Analysis of the Law in India by Ashish Chug and Satarupa Chakravortty

Para 3.1 of the National Guidelines states: Clinics involved in any one of the following activities should be regulated, licensed and supervised by the accreditation authority.

Para 3.5.3 of the National Guidelines states: The ART clinic must not be a party to any commercial element in donor programmes or in Gestational Surrogacy.

Para 3.10.3 of the National Guidelines states: Payments to Surrogate Mother should cover all genuine expenses associated with the pregnancy. Documentary evidence of the financial arrangement for surrogacy must be available.

The ART centre should not be involved in this monetary aspect.

Para 3.10.6 of the National Guidelines states: No relative or a person known to the couple may act as a Surrogate.

US

California Citations:

CAL. FAM. CODE § 7600 et seq. (2009).
Elisa B. v. Superior Court, 117 P.3d 660 (Cal. 2005).
Johnson v. Calvert, 851 P.2d 776 (Cal. 1993).
K.M. v. E.G., 117 P.3d 673 (Cal. 2005).
Kristine H. v. Lisa R., 117 P.3d 690 (Cal. 2005).
In re Marriage of Buzzanca, 72 Cal. Rptr. 2d 280 (Cal. Ct. App. 1998).
In re Marriage of Moschetta, 30 Cal. Rptr. 2d 893 (Cal. Ct. App. 1994).

Florida Citations

FLA. STAT. § 63.212 (2009).
FLA. STAT. §§ 742.11-16 (2009).
Lofton v. Kearney, 358 F. 3d 804 (11th Cir. 2004).
Lowe v. Broward County, 766 So. 2d 1199 (Fla. Dist. Ct. App. 2000).
Wakeman v. Dixon, 921 So. 2d 669 (Fla. Dist. Ct. App. 2006).

Bibliography

Appel, J.M., "China fears bachelor future." BBC News. April 5, 2004.

Beernink, FJ; Dmowski, WP; Ericsson, RJ (1993). "Sex preselection through albumin separation of sperm." *Fertility and sterility 59* (2): 382—6. PMID 8425635.

Boada, M.; Carrera, M.; De La Iglesia, C.; Sandalinas, M.; Barri, P. N.; Veiga, A. (1998). "Successful use of a laser for human embryo biopsy in preimplantation genetic diagnosis: report of two cases." *Journal of Assisted Reproduction and Genetics 15* (5): 302—7.doi:10.1023/A:1022548612107. PMID 9604764.

Bredenoord, Annelien; Dondorp, Wybo; Pennings, Guido; De Die-Smulders, Christine; Smeets, Bert; De Wert, Guido (2009). "Preimplantation genetic diagnosis for mitochondrial DNA disorders: ethical guidance for clinical practice." *European Journal of Human Genetics 17* (12): 1550—9.doi:10.1038/ejhg.2009.88. PMC 2987024. PMID 19471315.

Chen, M.; Guu, HF; Ho, ES (1997). "Efficiency of sex pre-selection of spermatozoa by albumin separation method evaluated by double-labelled fluorescence in-situ hybridization." *Human Reproduction 12* (9): 1920—6. doi:10.1093/humrep/12.9.1920.PMID 9363707.

Dmowski, WP; Gaynor, L; Rao, R; Lawrence, M; Scommegna, A (1979). "Use of albumin gradients for X and Y sperm separation and clinical experience with male sex preselection." *Fertility and sterility 31* (1): 52— PMID 283932.

Dugdale, David, M.D. (February 19, 2009). "Chromosome url=http://www.nlm.nih.gov/medlineplus/ency/article/002327.htm." U.S. National Library of Medicine.

Flegr, Jaroslav; Sulc, J; Nouzová, K; Fajfrlík, K; Frynta, D; Flegr, J (2007). "Women infected with parasite Toxoplasma have more sons," (PDF). Naturwissenschaften 94 (2): 122.doi:10.1007/s00114-006-0166-2. PMID 17028886.

Garner D.L., Seidel G.E. "History of commercializing sexed semen for cattle". *Theriogenology 2008*;69: 886-895.

Gray, R.H. (1991). "Natural family planning and sex selection: fact or fiction?" *American Journal of Obstetrics and Gynecology* 165 (6 Pt 2): 1982—4. PMID 1836712.

Hoag, Hannah. "I'll take a girl, please... Cherry-picking from the dish of life." Drexel University Publication.

Johnson, L. A., Flook, J. P., Look, M. V., Pinkel, D., "Flow sorting of X and Y chromosome-bearing spermatozoa into two populations". *Gamete Research Volume 16*, Issue1, pages 1-9, January 1987.

Johnson, L. A., Flook, J. P., Look, M. V., "Flow cytometry of X and Y chromosome-bearing sperm for DNA using an improved preparation method and staining with Hoechst 33342". *Gamete Research Volume 17*, Issue 3, July 1987, Pages: 203—212.

Kanavakis, E; Traeger-Synodinos, J (2002). "Preimplantation genetic diagnosis in clinical practice." *Journal of Medical Genetics 39* (1): 6—11. doi:10.1136/jmg.39.1.6. PMC 1734958.PMID 11826017.

Mayor, S. (2001). "Specialists question effectiveness of sex selection technique." *BMJ 323*: 67.doi: 10.1136/bmj.323.7304.67.

Pehlivan, T; Rubio, C; Rodrigo, L; Romero, J; Remohi, J; Simón, C; Pellicer, A (2003). "Impact of preimplantation genetic diagnosis on IVF outcome in implantation failure patients." *Reproductive BioMedicine Online 6* (2): 232—7. doi:10.1016/S1472-6483(10)61715-4. PMID 12676006.

Puri S, Nachtigall RD (May 2010). "The ethics of sex selection: a comparison of the attitudes and experiences of primary care physicians and physician providers of clinical sex selection services." Fertil. Steril. 93 (7): 2107—14.doi:10.1016/j.fertnstert.2009.02.053. PMID 19342036.

Rice, Mary. "Children born after PGD as healthy as those born after conventional IVF treatment." *European Society of Human Genetics*. Retrieved February 12, 2011.

Seidel G.E., Jr., Garner D.L. "Current status of sexing mammalian spermatozoa". *Reproduction 2002*;124: 733-743.

Shettles, L.; D.M. Rorvick (2006). "How Do They Compare?" In Martin J. Whittle and C. H. Rodeck. *How to Choose the Sex of Your Baby: The Method Best*

Supported by Scientific Evidence. New York: Random House. p. [1]. ISBN 978-0767926102.

Silverman, M.D., Ph.D., Andrew Y. "Gender Selection Ericsson Method". Retrieved February 13, 2011.

Silverman, M.D., Ph.D., Andrew Y. "Determine baby gender with IVF/PGD." Retrieved February 12, 2011.

US Patent 5,021,244, column 9, Sorting Sperm; http://patft.uspto.gov/netacgi/nph-Parser?Sect1=PTO1& Sect2=HITOFF&d=PALL&p=1&u=%2Fnetahtml%2FPTO %2Fsrchnum.htm&r=1&f=G&l=50&s1=5021244.PN.&OS =PN/5021244&RS=PN/5021244

US Patent 5,021,244; 5,346,990; 5,369,012; 5,439,362; 5,496,722; 5,648,468; 5,660,997; PCT/US1989/002069

Wilcox, Allen J. M.D., Ph.D., Weinberg, Clarice R., Ph.D., and Baird, Donna D., Ph.D. "Timing of Sexual Intercourse in Relation to Ovulation — Effects on the Probability of Conception, Survival of the Pregnancy, and Sex of the Baby," *N Engl J Med* 1995; 333:1517-1521 December 7, 1995.

Ancient Chinese birth gender chart.

China facing major gender imbalance, MSNBC, 12 Jan 2007. Archive http://web.archive.org/web/20080207012108/ http://www.msnbc.msn.com/id/16593301/

Foods That Harm, Foods That Heal', p. 203-204, by *Readers Digest*, 2004.

"India's lost girls," BBC Online, 4 Feb 2003.

"Infanticide, Abortion Responsible for 60 Million Girls Missing in Asia." Fox News. June 13, 2007.

"MicroSort Information." MicroSort, Inc.. Retrieved February 13, 2011.

"Sisters 'make people happy', US clinic offers British couples the chance to choose the sex of their child" from *The Times*. August 22, 2009.

"Want a Daughter? Try Paying for Her," *Opposing Views*, August 26, 2009.